A Field Guide to Type 1 Diabetes

The Essential Resource from the Diabetes Experts

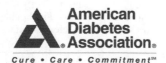

American Diabetes Association

Cure • Care • Commitment℠

Editor, Marie McCarren; *Director, Book Publishing*, John Fedor; *Associate Director, Consumer Books*, Sherrye Landrum; *Production Manager*, Peggy M. Rote; *Composition*, Circle Graphics, Inc.; *Cover Design*, Design Literate, Inc.; *Printer*, Transcontinental Printing

Printed in Canada
1 3 5 7 9 10 8 6 4 2

ADA titles may be purchased for business or promotional use or for special sales. To purchase this book in large quantities, or for custom editions of this book with your logo, contact Lee Romano Sequeira, Special Sales & Promotions, at the address below, or at LRomano@diabetes.org or 703-299-2046.

American Diabetes Association
1701 North Beauregard Street
Alexandria, Virginia 22311

Library of Congress Cataloging-in-Publication Data

A field guide to type 1 diabetes.
    p. cm.
  Includes index.
  ISBN 1-58040-170-8 (pbk. : alk. paper)
    1. Diabetes—Popular works. I. Title: Field guide to type one diabetes. II. American Diabetes Association.

RC660.4 .F545 2002
362.1′96462—dc21   2002026118

Contents

Acknowledgments

We thank Susan McLaughlin, BS, RD, CDE; David S. Schade, MD; and Donald K. Zettervall, RPH, CDE, for their careful review of this book.

This book contains material from case studies and articles that appeared in *Diabetes Forecast*. Contributors include Marjorie Cypress, RN, CDE; Dianne Davis, RD, CDE; Peggy Deitz, FNP, RN; Janie Lipps, RN, CDE; and Robert M. Mordkin, MD. We thank the staff of *Diabetes Forecast*, including Melody Merin, editor of the Reflections essays, and John C. Warren for technical assistance.

Introduction

One day, your life changed. On that day, you learned you had type 1 diabetes.

You may be recently diagnosed, or it may be old hat to you. In either case, your concern is the same: a high quality of life.

Good blood glucose control contributes a great deal to your quality of life—now and in the future.

Your doctor can prescribe insulin for you, your dietitian can advise you about food choices that help glucose control, your diabetes educator can help you choose which times are best for shots and exercise, but how you use this information to manage your diabetes is up to you. With diabetes, the person who has it is in charge from day to day.

You may want to take charge of your type 1 diabetes in steps. You might choose to learn more about how insulin works. Then maybe you'll want to work toward getting more flexible about when you eat and work out.

A Field Guide to Type 1 Diabetes gives you information for every step. It will help you make positive, life-affirming choices about your diabetes care.

Biology of Type 1 Diabetes

What Is Diabetes?

Diabetes is a group of diseases in which there is too much glucose (a kind of sugar) in the blood. Today, many types of diabetes are known. The two most common forms of the disease are:

- type 2 diabetes. People with type 2 diabetes use diet and exercise, pills, or insulin to control their disease. Most cases of diabetes are type 2 diabetes.
- type 1 diabetes. People with type 1 diabetes must use insulin. Type 1 diabetes affects less than 10% of all people with diabetes.

What Happened To Me?

We'll start before you developed type 1 diabetes.

Special cells in your pancreas, called beta cells, produced the hormone called insulin. Insulin helped glucose move from your bloodstream into your muscle and fat cells, and those cells used glucose for energy.

Your pancreas secreted insulin at a low level all day long. When you ate, the starches and sugars from the meal were broken down into glucose. The glucose moved into the bloodstream. Your pancreas secreted more insulin to take care of the extra glucose. Your blood glucose levels stayed in the range of 70–110 mg/dl before meals and not more than 140 mg/dl after meals.

Then you began to develop diabetes. Long before you were diagnosed, perhaps years before, your immune system started to attack the beta cells of your pancreas. Normally, the immune system attacks only foreign cells, such as bacteria and viruses. When it attacks the body's own cells, it's called an autoimmune process.

Some of your beta cells were destroyed by this autoimmune attack, but you had plenty of others left to do the work.

The destructive process continued. When most of your beta cells were destroyed, your body started having a little trouble dealing with glucose, but you still didn't have symptoms.

Then your body might have been put under stress. It could have been an illness, such as the flu. It could have been an emotional stress.

When you're under stress, your body wants you to have extra glucose available to

STATISTICS

There are about 123,000 children (younger than age 20) with type 1 diabetes in the U.S.

Peak incidence of type 1 diabetes is around 10–12 years old in girls and 12–14 years old in boys. There is a smaller peak around age 5 in boys.

About 30,000 Americans develop type 1 diabetes each year.

Type 1 diabetes is more common in whites than in African Americans, Hispanic Americans, or Asian Americans. Type 1 diabetes is rare in Native Americans.

There are an estimated 850,000– 1.7 million people with type 1 diabetes in the United States today.

Approximately one in every 400–500 children and adolescents has type 1 diabetes.

In both northern and southern hemispheres the incidence of the onset of type 1 diabetes is reduced during the summer.

help your body deal with the stress. It produces stress hormones, and one effect is that the liver releases stored glucose. This worked fine before you were developing diabetes— your beta cells simply put out more insulin so the body could use the extra glucose.

But by this time, most of your beta cells had been destroyed. Your few remaining beta cells could handle a normal amount of glucose, but they couldn't cover this extra glucose. Your blood glucose level went up.

High levels of glucose smother beta cells. Your remaining beta cells were still alive, but they stopped working. Your blood glucose level jumped even higher, and you noticed the symptoms of diabetes: You needed to urinate frequently and were very thirsty. You may have lost weight even though you were hungrier than usual and eating more. You felt tired, and your vision might have been blurry.

(The illness or emotional stress didn't cause your diabetes. It may have just made it show up a little earlier.)

Once you were diagnosed, you started to take insulin by injection. Your blood glucose levels came down. Freed of the excess glucose, your remaining beta cells came coughing back to life. They started to produce insulin again. You needed less injected insulin, and your blood glucose levels were easy to control. This is called the honeymoon period. It may have lasted weeks or months.

But the immune destruction of your beta cells continued. Eventually, all your beta cells were destroyed. Now all your insulin needs have to be met with injected insulin.

Why Me?

Through research, we are learning why diabetes develops.

STATISTICS

Estimated Risk of Developing Type 1 Diabetes

No diabetes in family	1% chance of type 1 diabetes by age 50

One parent with type 1
(risk is ~2 times higher if parent was diagnosed before age 11)

▩ Father	6% chance of type 1 diabetes
▩ Mother who was	
• under 25 years old at child's birth	4% chance of type 1 diabetes
• 25 or older at child's birth	1% chance of type 1 diabetes
Sibling with type 1 diabetes	10% chance of type 1 diabetes by age 50
Identical twin with type 1 diabetes	25–50% chance of type 1 diabetes

Genes, the basic units of heredity, clearly play a role in making some people more likely to get diabetes. Relatives of someone with type 1 diabetes have a higher risk for developing diabetes than nonrelatives.

Scientists have studied identical twins to find out how big a role genetics plays in diabetes. The genes of identical twins are the same. In sets of twins in which one has type 1 diabetes, the other twin also gets the disease at most only 25% to 50% of the time. This is 100 times the risk of the average American developing diabetes, so genes do increase a person's risk for diabetes.

Yet, even when they have genes putting them at risk, half or more of the co-twins never get type 1 diabetes. This shows that environment also plays a big role. At least 85% of people who develop type 1 diabetes have no known family history of type 1 diabetes, and that supports the role of environment in the process.

Parents of people with type 1 diabetes have a 5% risk of getting the disease. Siblings who aren't identical twins have a 7% to 10% risk. Children of those with type 1 diabetes have between a 1% and 6% risk. However, a child's risk is influenced by which parent has type 1 diabetes. Children are more likely to develop type 1 diabetes when their father has diabetes than when their mother does (see box on p. 5).

Taking all these associations together, it seems that a person who develops type 1 diabetes starts with a genetic susceptibility, and then has the misfortune to encounter some factor that triggers the start of the disease. Some of the suggested triggers are certain viruses and cow's milk. (Breastfed babies are less likely to develop diabetes than formula-fed babies).

CHAPTER 2

Insulin

A healthy pancreas puts out a low, steady stream of insulin day and night. This is called basal, baseline, or background insulin. The pancreas secretes extra insulin in response to meals (Figure 2-1).

You can recreate this (somewhat) with injections of different insulins (Figure 2-2). Glargine (Lantus) is a peakless long-acting insulin that provides basal insulin coverage.

Figure 2-1. Insulin Levels in a Person Who Doesn't Have Diabetes

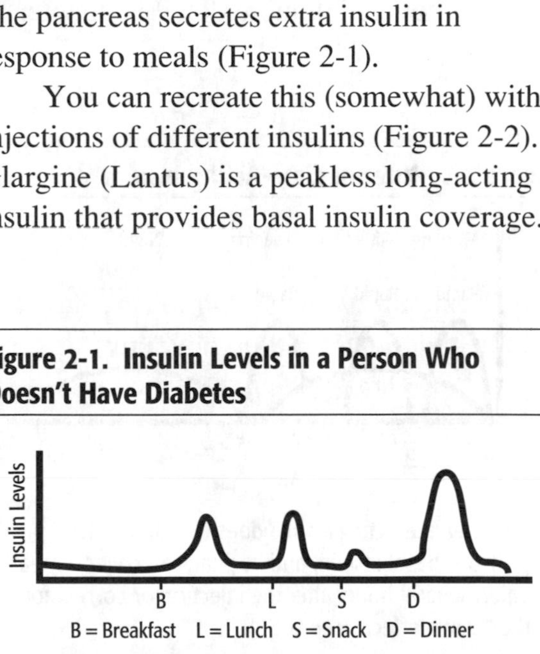
Insulin Levels
B
L
S
D
B = Breakfast L = Lunch S = Snack D = Dinner

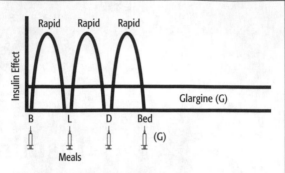

Figure 2-2. One Insulin Plan: Rapid Acting Plus Long Acting

Short- and rapid-acting insulins cover meals. Long-acting insulin covers basal needs.

By taking two kinds of insulin, for example rapid acting before each meal and long acting at bedtime, you can get close to normal insulin coverage (Figure 2-3). Insulin plans are covered in more detail in chapter 4.

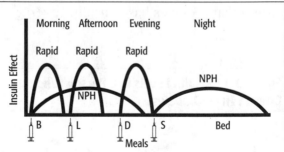

Figure 2-3. Intermediate-Acting Insulin

Intermediate-acting insulin does two things: It provides basal insulin, and its peak can cover a meal eaten several hours after the injection or correct for the "Dawn effect" (see p. 50).

Action Times

Three characteristics of insulin are important to know:

▨ **Onset.** The length of time before insulin reaches the bloodstream and begins lowering blood glucose.
▨ **Peak time.** The time during which insulin is working hardest in terms of lowering blood glucose levels.
▨ **Duration.** The total time the insulin lowers blood glucose.

Each person has his or her unique response to insulin, so the times in Table 2-1 are approximate. Only blood glucose checks will tell you how your body responds.

Types of Insulin

If you were diagnosed in recent years, you're probably using "human" insulin or an insulin analog.

Human insulin is made in labs. The human genetic code for insulin is inserted into bacteria or yeast, fooling them into producing insulin. Because bacteria and yeast multiply rapidly, they can produce large amounts of insulin. This technology allows us an almost unlimited supply of insulin to meet the growing demands.

Insulin analogs—aspart, glargine, and lispro—are like natural human insulin but with small changes that result in different action profiles. Insulin analogs require a prescription from your doctor.

Table 2-1. Insulins by Comparative Actions

Insulin Type	Onset	Peak (hours)	Usual Effective Duration (hours)	Usual Maximum Duration (hours)
Rapid-acting				
Aspart	5–10 minutes	1–3	3–5	4–6
Lispro	less than 15 minutes	0.5–1.5	2–4	4–6
Short-acting				
Regular	0.5–1 hour	2–3	3–6	6–10
Regular, pork	0.5–2 hours	3–4	4–6	6–8
Intermediate-acting				
NPH	2–4 hours	4–10	10–16	14–18
NPH, pork	4–6 hours	8–14	16–20	20–24
Lente	3–4 hours	4–12	12–18	16–20
Lente, pork	4–6 hours	8–14	16–20	20–24
Long-acting				
Ultralente	6–10 hours	10–16	18–20	20–24
Glargine	1 hour	no peak	24+	24+

Pork insulin is isolated from the pancreases of slaughterhouse pigs. Pork insulin is almost identical to human insulin. Although pork insulin is purified, it is more likely to cause an immune reaction than human insulin. Your body's immune system goes into action when anything foreign enters. Naturally, human insulin looks less foreign to your body than insulin from a pig.

If you're still using pork insulin (the three Iletin insulins in Table 2-2), you might consider switching to human insulin unless you have a known allergy to human insulin. Never change your type of insulin without consulting your doctor.

Rapid-acting Insulins: Newer, Faster, Better

Until the mid-1990s, regular insulin was the only short-acting insulin available. Regular isn't the perfect mealtime insulin, though.

It takes only about 10 minutes for food that you eat to start to be digested, absorbed, and to turn up as glucose in your blood. But it takes about 30 minutes after injection for regular insulin to start to lower blood glucose. If you inject regular insulin right before you eat, insulin action lags behind the rise in blood glucose, and your blood glucose levels will go too high until the insulin catches up. To get good coverage of a meal, you need to take regular 15–45 minutes before you start to eat, depending on your premeal blood glucose level (Table 2-3).

Most people find it inconvenient to have to take insulin so long before a meal. There

Table 2-2. Insulin Products

Product	Manufacturer/Distributor
Rapid-acting	
Humalog (lispro) * +	Lilly
NovoLog (aspart) *	Novo Nordisk
Short-acting (regular)	
Humulin R	Lilly
Iletin II Regular (pork)	Lilly
Novolin R * +	Novo Nordisk
Novolin BR (buffered)	Novo Nordisk
ReliOn/Novolin R	Wal-Mart (Novo Nordisk)
Intermediate-acting	
Humulin L (lente)	Lilly
Humulin N (NPH) +	Lilly
Iletin II Lente (pork)	Lilly
Iletin II NPH (pork)	Lilly
Novolin L (lente)	Novo Nordisk
Novolin N (NPH) * +	Novo Nordisk
ReliOn/Novolin N (NPH)	Wal-Mart (Novo Nordisk)
Long-acting	
Humulin U (ultralente)	Lilly
Lantus (glargine)	Aventis
Mixtures	
Humulin 50/50 (50% NPH, 50% regular)	Lilly
Humulin 70/30 (70% NPH, 30% regular)	Lilly
Humalog Mix 75/25 + (75% lispro protamine, 25% lispro)	Lilly
Novolin 70/30 * + (70% NPH, 30% regular)	Novo Nordisk
ReliOn/Novolin 70/30	Wal-Mart (Novo Nordisk)

* Also comes in pen cartridges.
+ Also comes in prefilled pens.

Table 2-3. Action to Take Based on Blood Glucose Level when You Use Regular Insulin

If blood glucose 45 minutes before meal is:	Right away:	Inject regular insulin:
Below 50	eat or drink something with sugar	when finishing the meal
50–70	eat or drink something with sugar	at mealtime
70–120		15 minutes before the meal
120–180		30 minutes before the meal
Over 180		45 minutes before the meal

are now two insulins that start to work more quickly and peak sooner than regular insulin: aspart (brand name NovoLog) and lispro (Humalog). Typically, you take them right before you eat. This is much more convenient, and it becomes even more important in certain situations:

■ **When you don't know when the food will come.** This is par for the course at restaurants. If you're on a plane, the food cart could be one row from you when the plane hits turbulence. With rapid-acting insulin, you can take your dose when the food is in front of you and not sacrifice good control.

■ **With children.** It's hard to predict how much a child will eat. If you give insulin before the meal and your child refuses to eat, you're put in the position of offering anything with sugar to protect against an insulin reaction. So parents are generally advised to wait until their child completes a meal and dose according to how much was eaten. Rapid-acting insulin acts quickly enough to cover the meal.

Even if your child is a good eater, rapid-acting insulin makes life easier. When your child says, "I'm hungry," he doesn't want to hear, "OK, here's your insulin. And now you have to wait a half-hour."

■ **You have gastroparesis.** Diabetes some-times causes nerve damage. When the nerves in the stomach are affected, food moves through the stomach slowly and unpredictably. You can check your blood glucose after you eat and when it starts to rise, take a rapid-acting insulin to cover the meal.

However, if you can't monitor your blood glucose after meals, you're proba-bly better off taking regular insulin. Its later peak and longer duration may more closely match your food's slow passage.

If You Switch from Regular Insulin to Rapid-Acting Insulin (lispro or aspart):

■ **Watch your "low" feelings.** Some peo-ple find that rapid-acting insulins drop their blood glucose level so quickly that they get symptoms of low blood glucose even when blood glucose isn't really low. Check your blood glucose level to be sure.

■ **Watch the carbohydrate content of your meal.** Say you're having fish and salad for dinner. There's very little starch there to turn into glucose. If you take a rapid-acting insulin before the meal, you'll likely get slammed by a "low" about an hour or so after the meal. See p. 81 for more on balancing carbohydrates and insulin.

Your doctor may want you to start out with a dose of rapid-acting insulin that is 10–15% lower than your old dose of regular. For a couple of weeks, check your blood glucose levels about 2 hours after the first bite of a meal to see if the rapid-acting insulin is bringing your blood glucose to the levels you want.

Mixed Insulins

You may be instructed to mix insulins. For example, if your insulin plan calls for two kinds of insulin in the morning, you may be able to mix the insulins in the syringe and take just one shot.

NPH insulin mixes easily with regular insulin. If need be, you can fill the syringes up to a week in advance.

You can also mix NPH with aspart or lispro, but you should inject the insulins right after you mix them.

Some doctors advise against mixing with lente or ultralente. Mixing may lead to unpredictable blood glucose results. However, some people have gotten good control with some of these mixtures. If your doctor suggests you mix lente or ultralente with another insulin, be sure to take the injection right after mixing it. Problems are more likely if the mixture is allowed to sit.

Lantus (Glargine) can NOT be mixed with any other insulin.

If it fits your insulin needs, you can use premixed insulins. (See Mixtures in Table 2-2.) These are helpful if you have trouble drawing up insulin out of two different bottles. Their disadvantage is that you can't change the doses independently of each other to fine-tune your control.

Insulin Strength

As long as you're buying insulin in the United States, you don't have to worry about different strengths of insulin. The strength available here is U-100. This means it has 100 units of insulin per milliliter of liquid.

Only one insulin is available in the U-500 mix (Humulin R, which also comes in U-100), but only by prescription and special order. It's used by those who develop insulin resistance and require extremely high doses of insulin.

U-40 is used in Latin America and Europe. It has 40 units of insulin per milliliter.

Insulin syringes also come in different sizes to match the strength of insulin. If you travel outside of the United States, bring along enough insulin and matching U-100 syringes. If you don't match insulin strength with the right size syringe, you can end up taking the wrong dose. If you plan a long stay out of the country and can't bring all the supplies you need, remember that the U-40 insulin found in Latin America and Europe will require a U-40 syringe. Your doctor or pharmacist can help you adjust your dosage.

Additives

All insulins have added ingredients. These prevent bacteria from growing and help keep the insulin from spoiling. Some intermediate- and long-acting insulins also contain ingredients that prolong their action times. Rarely, these additives, such as the protamine in NPH, cause allergic reactions. If you develop a rash or irritation every time you inject, talk to your doctor.

Buying Insulin

It pays to shop around. Prices for insulin may vary by several dollars per bottle. You may receive a discount for buying certain quantities at your pharmacy or by mail order.

If you want to order by mail, consider the effect of shipping during hot summer months in the South or freezing winter months in the North. Ask the distributor how the bottles are kept cool and inspect the bottles when they arrive.

Your insurance company may have a relationship with a "preferred pharmacy" or insulin manufacturer, which can change from time to time. If a change is necessary remember to tell your doctor and check your blood sugars more often just in case your dose needs to be adjusted.

When buying insulin (especially if you are buying in bulk), check the expiration date. Store the unopened bottles in the refrigerator and make sure you will use the insulin before it expires.

Develop a relationship with a professional pharmacist. Feel free to ask questions. If you consistently use the same pharmacist, he or she may be able to work directly with your doctor and advise you on insulin adjustments. The pharmacist can also let you know when a new insulin or injection device becomes available that could make management easier.

Consider choosing a pharmacy that is close by or one that delivers your insulin to you. Many people find they like the convenience of having their insulin delivered, especially if they are busy or ill.

Don't just ask for "NPH insulin." Look at the full brand name, strength, and kind. Bring along an empty bottle to make sure you get exactly the same thing each time. Before you pay, double check to see that you have what you want.

Remember, some insulins, such as Humalog, require a prescription. When you travel, bring one with you or bring the prescription label from your pharmacy. This way if you run out, a pharmacist near you can contact your doctor or original pharmacy and get you what you need. If you fly, you must have a prescription or the medications with the prescription label on the box.

Storing Insulin

Store unopened bottles of insulin in the refrigerator whenever possible.

If you go through a bottle of insulin in about a month, you don't need to refrigerate it between injections. Injecting cold insulin can make the injection uncomfortable. Put a cold bottle of insulin in your pocket for a few minutes to warm it up before you draw out the insulin, or warm a filled syringe by holding it or gently rolling it between your hands.

Don't keep an open vial of insulin at room temperature for longer than about a month after you first puncture it. The insulin strength may decrease. If you go through bottles slowly, write the date you first use a new bottle on the label.

If you store insulin in a cooler when on a trip, make sure the bottle doesn't touch the ice or freeze. Insulin spoils if it gets colder than 36°F. Don't expose your insulin to heat (such as in the glove compartment) and don't let it sit in direct sun. Insulin spoils if it gets hotter than 86°F. The general rule of thumb is, if the temperature is comfortable for you, your insulin will be okay, too.

Generally manufacturers recommend that insulin in cartridges or pens not be used for longer than 10 or 14 days once you start to use them. Check the manufacturer's instructions or ask your pharmacist.

Normal Appearance

Never use insulin that looks abnormal. Regular, lispro, aspart, and glargine insulins are clear liquids. Check for particles or discoloration; any cloudiness may indicate contamination and you should not use them.

Other types of insulin are suspensions. That means there is solid material floating in liquid. It should look uniformly cloudy. If you use NPH or lente, look for and avoid any insulin that has "frosting" inside the bottle or large clumps floating in it. These changes in the insulin mean crystals are forming. This can be caused by excessive shaking of the insulin, extremes of temperature, and improper zinc/insulin ratios.

If you find any of these things wrong with your insulin at the time of your purchase, return it immediately. If the condition develops later, try to determine if you have stored or handled the insulin the wrong way. If not, talk to your pharmacist about a refund or exchange.

FAITH HEALING

I was diagnosed with diabetes almost 40 years ago. Because my family was deeply religious and very involved with the church in our small east Tennessee town, diabetes instantly became a faith issue for me.

I remember sitting in front of the black-and-white T.V. set at my grandparents' house and watching religious programs. I'd see Oral Roberts performing healings and wondered what he could do with my diabetes. I often got on my knees at night and prayed for God to heal me and cure me of my diabetes. The next morning, I wondered if I should take my insulin. If I have faith that God heals, should I have faith not to take my shots? Practicality won out—I always took my insulin. But somehow, my faith was not thwarted.

Even as a child and later as an adolescent, I figured that God would work in God's own time. If and when I was healed, I would know it. Meanwhile, I prayed for doctors and researchers to find a cure.

By the time I was able to live on my own, disposable needles and syringes were available. I took one shot a day, until I realized that the amount of insulin I took was causing greater discomfort than the needle. Once I started two shots a day, it became much easier to go to three, four, or even five shots.

In college, I became a pre-ministerial student. From college to seminary, the faith issue kept recurring. I tried to explain to a small group of pastors one day that God's grace was sufficient for me to live with my diabetes. A few minutes later, two of them cornered me. "When you are ready, Tom," said one of them, "we'll anoint you with oil and get rid of that disease." My residual anger toward God for having the disease in the first place was kindled toward these well-intentioned but terribly insensitive colleagues.

While in seminary, I met with a group of students and laity to discuss faith and prayer. When it became known that I was diabetic, someone asked if the group could pray for my healing. The group had a warm and gentle spirit so I readily agreed.

At an appointed time, I sat in a chair in the middle of a circle. Members of the group—15 to 20 in number—laid their hands on me and prayed.

Some prayed audibly, some silently, some individually, and some together. All prayed for my healing. The outpouring of love felt good, even though no dramatic change occurred.

Later, as we left the building, a man said to me, "Now, Tom, don't take any more insulin. God has healed you. You've got to claim it." A kind woman heard this and said to me, "Tom, go ahead and take your insulin. It may not have been tonight, but God will heal you and you will know when it happens." Another man told me, "Don't worry. We'll all be healed in the resurrection."

That was over 20 years ago, when I had been diabetic a little less than 20 years. I registered their comments and I knew then, as I know now, that God had healed me. God healed me as I learned to accept the fact that I was diabetic and as I learned to live responsibly with it.

The issues of faith and of life and death have this in common: We must learn to accept the things we cannot change, accept them without blame and despair. We must work to change the things we can. This takes patience and perseverance. As the familiar prayer says, "God, grant me the wisdom to know the difference."

Thomas M. Reed
Diabetes Forecast
December 2000

Insulin Delivery: Where and How

Four areas have enough tissue under the skin for insulin injection (Figure 3-1):

- **Upper arm.** Inject into the outer back part of the upper arms where there is fatty tissue.
- **Abdomen.** Anywhere in the abdomen except within an inch of the navel, which has tough tissue that causes erratic absorption.
- **Thighs.** Tops and outside. Avoid the inner thighs because rubbing may make the injection site sore.
- **Buttocks.**

Insulin is absorbed and starts working most consistently when it's injected into the abdomen. When an arm, thigh, or buttock is used, how fast the insulin is absorbed and begins working will depend on how much

Figure 3-1. Locations for Insulin Injections

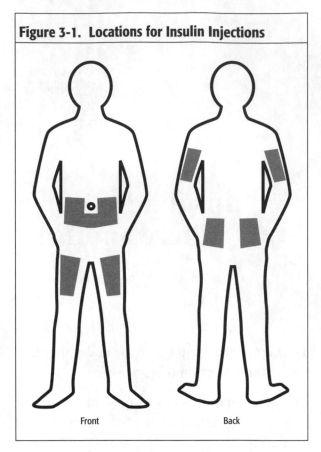

Front   Back

you use the muscles in the area after you inject.

Rapid-acting insulin analogs start working so quickly that generally it doesn't matter what site you choose. However, the site you choose can affect absorption of longer-acting insulins, so don't choose a site at random. If you choose your abdomen for your breakfast shot one day and you choose your thigh the next morning, you may get very different results. Instead, inject into the same body part at the same time of day.

Be aware that anything that affects blood flow to the area will affect absorption. Exercise increases blood flow, so some experts advise not injecting into an area that you will be strenuously exercising within 30 minutes. For example, you may want to avoid injecting in your thigh if you're going to go biking.

If you have a fever, are hot, or have been in a sauna, blood flow to your skin is increased, and absorption will be quicker. Smoking reduces blood flow, so try not to smoke within an hour before or after an injection.

Whatever site you choose, if you inject too often into the same spot in your skin, you may develop skin problems. You may get a build-up of fat, which makes the skin look lumpy. These lumps also slow absorption.

Although more rare, it is also possible to get a breakdown of the fatty tissue at an injection site if it is used too frequently, especially if you use pork insulin. This leads to depressions in the skin, which can also cause more erratic insulin absorption.

To avoid skin problems, inject at least a finger's width away from your last injection. Don't go back to any one spot for at least a week, and longer if you use an insulin pump.

Don't inject near moles or scar tissue.

Needles and Syringes

Most people use the standard needle-and-syringe method to get insulin into their bodies. Today you can find needles that are slimmer, have sharper points, and are specially coated to slide into the skin smoothly. These improvements help make your injections practically painless. Disposable syringes with lubricated microfine needles will give the smoothest penetration of your skin and will be the most comfortable. If your injections are still painful, review your injection technique with your doctor or diabetes educator. Learn to relax before you inject yourself. Tense muscles can make the injection hurt.

Keep your risk of infection low by making sure your injection site is clean. Good hygiene is all you need. You can use an alcohol pad to wipe the area first if you feel it needs it. However, this doesn't mean you have to use alcohol to clean your injection site every time, and never wipe the needle with alcohol. This will remove the lubrication on the needle and make it hurt more. See p. 179 for tips on preparing an insulin injection.

Buying Syringes

For U-100 insulin, you need U-100 syringes. Your other consideration is syringe size and readability. Your syringe needs to be large enough to hold your entire dose but small enough to allow for the easiest reading of the marking scale. For example, if you need to take 17 units of insulin, use a 1/3 cc (30-unit) syringe. It will be much easier to measure the correct dose because each line equals 1 unit. If you used a 100 unit syringe each line is equal to 2 units and the lines are closer together making them harder to see.

- 1cc = 100 units, each line is 2 units
- 1/2cc = 50 units, each line is 1 unit
- 1/3cc = 30 units, each line is 1 unit

Can you read the markings on the syringe you currently use? You need to do this to get an accurate dose. If the syringe you're using is the correct size and you still have trouble seeing the markings, ask your pharmacist for a syringe magnifier (Magni-Guide). Not only does this device make the markings easier to read, it also holds the insulin bottle and makes drawing the insulin easier.

If you plan to be away from home, in addition to taking enough diabetes supplies, take along a doctor's prescription for syringes, medication in the original box with your prescription label, and perhaps a letter from him or her stating that you have diabetes and your insulin type. In some states, you may not be able to obtain your syringes without a prescription. If you run out, the local pharmacist can easily contact your physician or original pharmacy, but if you encounter problems getting your supplies while traveling, try a hospital emergency room.

Reusing Syringes

Deciding whether to use your syringe more than once is up to you. It's a money saver, and there's no evidence that reusing a properly maintained syringe increases your chance of infection. However, if you have poor personal hygiene, are ill, have open wounds on your hands, or have decreased resistance to infection for any reason, don't risk reusing syringes. If a needle touches anything other than clean skin, it might carry germs into your body, and it's time to throw it away. Each time you use a needle it takes some of the lubricant off the needle and the needle gets a little duller, which means it will hurt more each time you inject.

Pen needles should always be removed right after use. When left in place, insulin can leak out and air or foreign material can get in, which could contaminate your insulin.

Getting Rid of Syringes

Don't just toss an old syringe into the trash can. An accidental stick with your insulin syringe could give a stranger a lot of worry. Used syringes are medical waste and need proper disposal. Your town or county may have rules about disposing of needles and other medical waste such as lancets.

Removing the needle will prevent anyone from ever using the syringe again. Clipping needles off syringes is a first step only if you do it correctly. It's best to buy a device that clips, catches, and contains the needle. Don't use scissors to clip off needle tips—the flying needle could hurt someone or become lost until someone is accidentally stuck with it. Bending your needle is another way to destroy it, if you can do it safely. One way is to pull out the plunger, push the needle into the plunger, bend the needle, break it off, and reinsert the plunger with the needle into the syringe.

If you don't destroy your needles, recap them if you can do it safely. The best place is an official "Sharps Container" which you can buy at your local pharmacy.

If this isn't possible, place the needle or entire syringe in an opaque (not clear) heavy-duty plastic or metal container with a screw cap or other closure. Label the container "MEDICAL WASTE—USED SHARPS." Don't use a container that will allow a needle to break through and possibly stick someone. Place the container in the trash where it will not be confused with recycling.

Injection Aids

Talk with your doctor or diabetes educator about these products. Often, they can give you samples to try before you purchase any. The annual Resource Guide in *Diabetes Forecast* lists information and suppliers of different types of aids.

Insertion Aids

Do you hate to see the needle? Do you have arthritis or problems holding a syringe steady? An automatic injector may be for you. Hold it to your skin, push a button, and the spring-loaded device inserts a needle into your skin almost without your knowing it. Some automatically release the insulin when the needle enters the skin. With others, you have to press the plunger on the syringe.

Infusers

These reduce the number of times you have to pierce your skin. With a special needle, you insert an infusion tube into your abdomen. The tube remains in place at the injection site for two or three days. Insulin is injected into the tube, which reseals after each needle entry. Because these infusers are usually sold in boxes, ask your doctor whether you can try just one before you commit yourself to buying a whole box. There is an increased risk of infection with this aid, so you may have to learn how to keep your technique cleaner than usual.

Jet Injectors

Want to be free of needles altogether? Maybe the jet injector is for you. The insulin is shot out so fast that it acts like a liquid needle, passing directly through the skin.

A jet injector is expensive and often not covered by insurance. Check with your insurance company about coverage. Over time you could save the cost of needles and syringes, but it is a large initial cost. Most of these devices are also much larger than syringes and not as easy to carry with you.

Bruising is sometimes a problem, particularly with thin people, children, and the elderly. However, you can get a jet injector that delivers insulin at a lower pressure.

Ask your doctor and diabetes educator what their patients think of jet injectors. Be aware that you may find that your insulin is absorbed more quickly when you use a jet injector.

Pen Devices

An insulin pen looks just like an ink pen. It has a disposable needle instead of a writing point, and an insulin cartridge instead of an ink cartridge. A cartridge holds 150 or 300 units of insulin that can be delivered in the measured amounts you need. You "dial in" your dose (clicks and a number dial tell you how much you've dialed in), and then inject. These pens are popular because they're so convenient and accurate in dose. You don't have to worry about filling syringes ahead of time and carrying them with you when you're away from home. If you're in a dim restaurant, the clicks tell you how much you've drawn up.

Pens cost about $35 to $50. Few health plans cover pens. Check to see whether yours does, and whether a prescription is required for it to be covered. Keep your eyes peeled for promotions. Your pharmacist or doctor may have coupons—ask.

Aids for the Visually Impaired

Several products are available to make injections easier for people who are visually or physically impaired. They include:

- **Dose gauges** to help you measure your insulin accurately (even mixed doses). Some have an audible click with each 1–2 units of insulin, and others have Braille or raised numbers.
- **Needle guides** and vial stabilizers to help you insert the needle into the insulin vial correctly. A few of these also allow you to set a desired dosage level with a dial or other device.
- **Syringe magnifiers** to enlarge the measure marks on an insulin syringe barrel.

Insulin Pumps

An insulin pump is a computerized device about the size of a beeper that you can wear on your belt or in your pocket. Inside is a reservoir (which resembles a syringe or cartridge), filled with a two- to three-day supply of rapid- or short-acting insulin. An infusion set—thin plastic tubing—is connected to the reservoir. The other end of the tubing is inserted underneath your skin, usually at the abdomen or "pockets" area on the buttocks. You change the infusion set and use a new site every two to three days.

The pump delivers a low, steady dose of insulin all day long. The basal rate for pumps can be adjusted from 0.1–10.0 units per hour based on your needs. This takes the place of injections of long-acting insulin. Just before you eat, you program the pump to deliver a surge (bolus) of insulin to cover the meal. This takes the place of your premeal injection.

A major advantage of a pump is that it's always delivering a controlled amount of insulin. You don't have to worry about when a long-acting insulin will peak or the timing of injections or meals. You can also stop or change the amount of insulin being delivered at any time, such as when you exercise. The biggest advantage is you only have to fill the reservoir and change the infusion set every few days, so no more injections several times a day. You just push a button to give yourself your insulin before meals or any time you eat. You can do this anywhere, anytime.

There's even a pump with a remote control. You can control the pump without touching it. That means it can be worn under clothing. You can even take the pump off for an hour or two from time to time and still maintain control.

Some problems you can have with a pump: Clogged or kinked tubing may reduce insulin delivery and can cause ketoacidosis. The insertion site may get infected. Overuse of an insertion site can cause the same skin problems that injecting into the same sites does.

Experts disagree about whether children should be on insulin pumps, but there are more children being placed on pumps every year. If your child is young, your child will be the pump "wearer," you will be the pump "user"—you'll be making the decisions about bolus doses, checking the infusion site for infection, etc. If you're considering a pump for your child, you may be asked by your child's health care team to wear the pump first (with sterile saline instead of insulin). Some school-aged children only wear the pump at night and use injections during the day at school.

If your child is older—preteen or teen— it must be his or her decision whether to get a pump. Pump use requires a thorough understanding of carbohydrate counting and choosing the matching insulin doses. If your child gets a pump because you pushed the idea, he or she won't be committed to using it correctly, and that could lead to big problems.

Pumps cost about $5,000, and pump supplies cost about $1,500 a year. With a doctor's prescription, some insurance companies will cover some of the cost. Medicare also covers pumps in certain cases.

Your doctor or diabetes educator may have materials such as video tapes or brochures to help you decide whether a pump is right for you. Pumps are growing in popularity, however some doctors may not be familiar with or comfortable with pumps. Ask him or her first, then check with a diabetes educator or find out if there is a pump support group in your area. This is a great way to learn more about them.

Insulin Plans

Your purpose in taking insulin is to make up for a malfunctioning pancreas. It makes sense to put insulin into your body as close to the way a normal pancreas would. That means a low, steady stream of insulin day and night, and extra insulin after you eat.

How does your insulin regimen measure up? Would a new approach be better? Have a frank discussion with your health care team. They will help you choose a plan.

Instead of always saying "Everything is just fine," speak up if anything is bothering you. Is there a problem when you exercise? Are you afraid to take a job that might require more travel? Are you more tired than you think you should be? Maybe it's time for a change. Unless you bring up the possibility of change or mention problems with your blood glucose results, each member of your health care team may assume you are satisfied with things as they are.

Regimen: One Shot (Rating: 1/2*)

One shot of insulin a day, only one needle a day—it sounds too good to be true. And, it is. No single shot of insulin can give you the basal insulin you need throughout the day plus higher levels of insulin to cover meals.

Regimen: Two Shots a Day (Rating:**)

Some people take two shots a day: intermediate-acting plus short- or rapid-acting insulin in the morning and evening (Figure 4-1). The peak of the morning rapid-acting covers breakfast, the peak of the intermediate-acting covers lunch, the peak of the evening rapid-acting covers dinner, the intermediate-acting dose in the evening provides basal insulin throughout the night.

On a two-shot program, you have to eat your meals on a regular schedule. The inter-

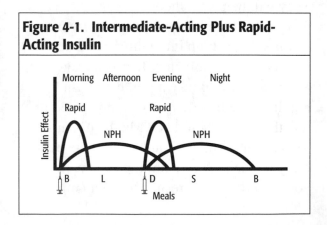

Figure 4-1. Intermediate-Acting Plus Rapid-Acting Insulin

mediate-acting insulin is going to peak at lunch time whether you want to eat then or not. You can't decide at the last minute to skip lunch. If lunch is delayed, you may have to eat a snack to keep from going low.

More important, a two-shot regimen lets you get only average—but usually not good—blood glucose control.

Want a plan that's more flexible and lets you get better blood glucose control? Read on.

Regimen: Flexible Insulin Plans (Rating: ****)

Flexible insulin plans mimic the normal insulin delivery that your pancreas provided before you had diabetes. You can use:

- **Three or more shots a day**: a long-acting insulin for basal coverage and rapid-acting insulin before each meal. A very good plan for many people is glargine at night and lispro or aspart before meals.
- **An insulin pump**, which delivers a slow trickle of insulin throughout the day and bolus doses to cover meals.

"We've been able to have some flexibility back in our lives. We can eat at seven rather than at six. That's a big deal."

—Stephanie Gosselin, whose husband is on a flexible insulin plan

These plans are flexible in three ways:

- **You can change your schedule.**
  Figure 4-2 shows a flexible insulin plan. You can vary the times of the mealtime

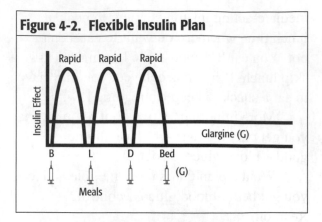

Figure 4-2. Flexible Insulin Plan

injections. You can wait until an office meeting breaks up to eat lunch. You can adapt if your school has rolling lunch times—you can eat lunch at 10:45 one day and 12 o'clock the next.

■ **You can change how much you eat.** You can eat more or less than you normally would—you just increase or decrease your mealtime insulin dose.

■ **You can fine-tune your control.** With flexible insulin plans, you check your blood glucose levels before meals and before bed. Then you can adjust your mealtime insulin doses according to the results using your sliding scale (see p. 46), correcting for lows or highs. This leads to better average blood glucose levels.

With an insulin pump, you can even have a flexible basal dose. For example, you can program the pump to always deliver less insulin around 2 a.m., reducing your risk of a low, and more insulin around 6 a.m., so you don't wake up with a morning high (see dawn phenomenon, p. 50).

"It's the one thing in 20 years of being diabetic that has allowed me the control to say, 'No, I don't feel like eating,' or 'Yes, I want to eat and this is what I want to eat.' It's allowed me a lot of freedom that I never had before."

—Theresa Kiwak, who switched to a flexible insulin plan

Flexible insulin plans do mean more work and expense. You'll be estimating the carb in your meal, using a sliding scale, and doing more blood glucose checks. When would that make sense for you? Ask yourself:

- Am I doing everything right yet still am not satisfied with my average blood glucose levels?
- Do I frequently have unexpected highs or lows?
- Do I have signs of the complications of diabetes?
- Do I lack the energy I need to participate in all my activities—both day and night?
- Do I want more flexibility in timing my meals, exercise, and other activities?

Careful Change

You can't start a flexible insulin plan on your own. You need information, instruction, and support. Ask your health care team about their experience with flexible insulin plans. It's possible that your doctor will feel more comfortable referring you to a diabetes specialist or to a diabetes care center that offers a complete management package.

Fast Food

Karen Briggs* was diagnosed with type 1 diabetes when she was 19. Her prescribed insulin regimen was two shots a day: a mixture of NPH and regular before breakfast and again before supper. Her dietitian recommended three balanced meals and two snacks a day.

Five years later, Ms. Briggs A1C's (see pp. 56–59) were 9% to 10% and her blood glucose results ranged from 40 mg/dl–350 mg/dl with no apparent pattern. She was angry about her poor control and frustrated about the rigid meal plan she was expected to follow.

Ms. Briggs went to see a nurse practitioner. She reported that she usually skipped breakfast. Lunch was fast food, but she sometimes skipped lunch too and just snacked. Some days she got off work at 3 p.m., other days she worked until 6 p.m. She sometimes ate a slice of pizza on the way home and ate supper later. Ms. Briggs hadn't told her doctor or her first dietitian what her schedule was like.

The nurse practitioner explained that there were insulin plans that would work with Ms. Briggs' unstructured lifestyle. But these plans would mean more shots and more blood glucose checks. Ms. Briggs was willing to make the commitment.

Ms. Briggs had two sessions with the nurse practitioner to learn about the new insulin plan (glargine for basal insulin, plus rapid-acting insulin before meals), and two appointments with a dietitian to learn carbohydrate counting.

There were also follow-up phone calls and faxes.

Four months later, Ms. Briggs' A1C was 6.9%, and she didn't have the extreme highs and lows she'd had before. She was much happier with her diabetes plan.

Names in the case studies have been changed.

Do you already have a dietitian and a diabetes educator who can help you learn the skills you need for a flexible plan? Your health care team will need to be committed to teaching you how to interpret your blood glucose checks and how to adjust your insulin, food, and activity.

Changing your insulin plan requires time and energy to make sure you're solving problems, not creating new ones. But the end result should make you feel better and fit the life you want to live. If you're trying a new approach, here are some questions to ask:

- How long will this type of insulin take to get into my bloodstream?
- When will it be most active?
- How long can I expect it to lower blood glucose?
- How will my choice of injection site affect absorption?
- Can I mix different types of insulin in one shot without affecting their action?
- How often and at what time of day should I inject my insulin?

Go step by step through this new insulin routine for a typical day with your doctor or nurse educator. Talk about how to adjust for an unusual day—oversleeping, illness, or travel. Write everything down. Compare what you expect with what actually happens to you.

THE LESSONS I'M LEARNING

I'm sure my doctor knew within 30 seconds that I had diabetes.

"I've lost 40 pounds in the last two months," I told him. "I feel tired all the time. My muscles are sore and tight. I urinate constantly, and I drink over a gallon of water a day." I didn't know until weeks later that I had been describing all the typical symptoms of diabetes. They could have been checked off a list one by one.

"You have diabetes," he said, as simply as he might have said, "You have strep." I believe that's why I responded, "For how long?"

This won't just go away? I don't take antibiotics for two weeks and get better?

When my doctor mentioned that many newly diagnosed patients are admitted to the hospital to start insulin therapy, I told him, "I have to go back to school. I have exams." I wasn't about to fall behind in my courses. I was insistent, and he agreed to work with me over the phone.

Of course I was in no shape to prepare for tests. I opened the books, read my notes, but all I could think about was my next injection. Life was a countdown from breakfast to lunch to dinner to bedtime. After a few days I knew that studying was hopeless, and the university excused me from taking my exams. Going back to school to take final exams just days after learning you have diabetes? What was I thinking?

After I became accustomed to taking injections, I thought the hardest part was behind me. I was mistaken. Injections were the easy part; you grow conditioned to four injections a day quicker than you might expect. But changing your understanding of food, stress, exercise—even the future itself—is not as simple, especially at the age of 20.

Nevertheless, after a few months, when I became comfortable testing my blood sugar, calculating the carbohydrate content of my meals, and adjusting my insulin, I thought I had essentially surmounted diabetes.

Again, what was I thinking?

I have had diabetes for eight years and have finally come to terms with the fact that I will never fully come to terms with diabetes. Strangely, this is more of a comfort to me now than a discouragement. I kept trying to reach the point at which everything would click into place and all of diabetes would become as mechanical as changing the cartridge of my insulin pen. Managing diabetes with ease and aplomb had become not just a goal but a test of self-respect, as if failure to take diabetes in stride were a character flaw. But I've realized there is no date on the calendar after which diabetes will become easy. It isn't easy. It never will be.

Diabetes made me think about the years ahead. The future is intangible, but I can feel myself creating that future with the decisions I make every day. The consequences are distant, but what determines those consequences could hardly be more immediate: Every meal, every injection, every blood sugar test is the raw material that my health is fashioned from. Life is just the sum of all the individual days.

These are things that my doctor could not have explained to me that day when he told me I had diabetes. I could never have seen then that I would never master diabetes like I mastered algebra in high school. Treating diabetes isn't one of those things you never forget how to do, like riding a bicycle. No matter how good my blood sugars were last week, I might fall off the bike this week. But I don't mind keeping the training wheels on and working at it a little each day.

David Ragsdale
Diabetes Forecast
June 2001

5

Checks and Balances

Life happens. One day you feel great so you swim a few extra laps. Another day your office mate brings in chocolate chip muffins. Then your usual lunchtime jog is replaced by a gotta-have-it-now report for your boss.

Life is reflected in your blood glucose results. When you check your blood glucose level before a meal, you'll often get results that are higher or lower than your goal range.

Even if you keep your food intake and activity exactly the same from day to day, there are things you can't control. For example, how much insulin your body absorbs can vary by as much as 25% from day to day. This is especially true of NPH insulin. So expect the unexpected result.

Do you just have to shrug and do nothing? No—you can take action to correct for those out-of-range numbers.

How Much

If you take rapid- or short-acting insulin before meals, you can correct for highs and lows by changing how much insulin you take. You follow an insulin "sliding scale" (also called a supplemental insulin scale) worked out for you by your health care team. Before you take a mealtime shot, you check your blood glucose level. If it's high, you take a little more mealtime insulin; if it's low you take a little less.

The first step toward using a sliding scale is for you and your health care provider to work out your blood glucose goals. These depend on your age, other medical conditions, and other variables such as the kind of work you do.

Next, a sliding scale is prescribed for you. It depends on how sensitive to insulin you are. This is affected by your weight (thin people are usually more sensitive to insulin than people who are overweight) and your age (adolescents are less sensitive to insulin than adults or children).

Here is one example: Ms. Beranek is 22 years old. She uses glargine for basal coverage and lispro before meals. Her blood glucose goal before meals is 70–130 mg/dl. Her diabetes educator has figured out a sliding scale for her. If Ms. Beranek's blood glucose before a meal is 70–130 mg/dl, she takes her usual dose of lispro based on the carb she ate. If her blood glucose is 130–150 mg/dl,

she increases her lispro 1 unit. If it's
150–200 mg/dl, she takes an extra 2 units of
lispro. If Ms. Beranek's blood glucose is low
before the meal, she takes less lispro.

When

You can also correct for highs and lows by
changing when you take your mealtime
insulin. If you use aspart or lispro, you usually take your insulin right before you start to
eat. When your premeal blood glucose is
below 70 mg/dl, your sliding scale may have
you delay your shot until after you start eating, in addition to reducing the dose. For the
timing of regular insulin, see p. 13.

Pattern Management

You check your blood glucose before lunch
and it's a little high. No problem. You use
your sliding scale to correct for it. The next
day at lunch, it's a little high again. Again
you use your sliding scale to correct for it.
Third day: high again before lunch.

"You know yourself better than anyone, you know
what's happening with your life, and you can regulate
your blood sugars to feel your best."
**—Laurie Carson, who uses pattern management to
fine-tune her insulin plan**

You start to wonder, Can't I do something to *prevent* these out-of-range levels
instead of just reacting to them after the fact?
Yes, you can. It's called pattern management. A pattern is when:

■ your blood glucose is high at the same time of day three days in a row

■ your blood glucose is low at the same time two days in a row

When you see a pattern, identify which insulin is active at the time of the high or low. (Review Table 2-1, p. 10.) The next day you change the insulin to prevent the high or low. You change the dose by only 1 or 2 units at a time (ask your health care team). Make little corrections.

You can also watch for patterns over a longer period of time. That pattern of lows two Tuesdays in a row? Probably because you started playing racquetball on Tuesdays. Maybe you have seasonal patterns: higher glucose levels in the winter that come back down in the spring when you come out of hibernation.

Pattern management helps you fine-tune your plan to fit your changing needs. To do pattern management, you need:

■ **A willingness to check.** You'll need to check your blood glucose level four times a day.

■ **Blood glucose goals.** Work these out with your health care team.

■ **An accurate meter.** Check your meter with a control strip. Ask your health provider to check your technique and to check your results against lab results.

■ **A blood glucose log.** Check your blood glucose before meals and before bed. Write down the results (see p. 202). You may want to highlight highs in one color and lows in another color so you can see patterns more easily.

Soccer Days

Jacob is 8 years old. He takes NPH and a rapid-acting insulin in the morning and before supper.

Jacob recently joined a soccer team that practices after school. The first day of practice, his blood glucose was low at supper (60 mg/dl). His father reduced his usual rapid-acting meal-time insulin by 2 units, according to Jacob's sliding scale. Jacob's blood glucose was also low at bedtime (100 mg/dl), so he ate an extra snack.

The next day, Jacob was again low before supper and before bed. The NPH that Jacob takes in the morning is peaking in the afternoon. So on the third morning, his mother gave Jacob a little less NPH, according to instructions their doctor had given them at Jacob's last check-up. That day at supper and bedtime, Jacob's blood glucose levels were in his goal range. So his mother uses the new NPH morning dose on soccer days and the old NPH dose on days that Jacob doesn't have soccer.

■ **Instruction from your health care team.** You'll need their help on what to do when you see a pattern.

Morning Highs

Do you see a pattern of highs when you wake up in the morning? To find out what's causing them, check your blood glucose two nights in a row between 2 a.m. and 3 a.m. and again at 7 a.m. The table on the following page may help.

Table 5-1. Morning Highs

If your blood glucose at 2 a.m. to 3 a.m. is:	The cause might be:	Possible solution:
Higher than your bedtime glucose and even higher by morning	Too little insulin active during the night	Increase your intermediate- or long-acting insulin at supper or bedtime
Low	When faced with a low, the body releases hormones that raise blood glucose, and you may see a rebound high blood glucose by morning. (There is some controversy about how much rebounding contributes to morning highs.)	Lower your intermediate- or long-acting insulin at supper or bedtime. Talk to your health care team about programming your pump to deliver less insulin in the middle of the night.
About the same as it was at bedtime but is much higher by morning	The dawn phenomenon. In the early morning hours, certain hormones increase. These raise blood glucose levels. To counteract this, you need more basal insulin from about 4 a.m. to 8 a.m. In contrast, you naturally need less insulin from about 1 a.m. to 3 a.m.	Move your intermediate-acting insulin from suppertime to bedtime. This pushes the peak closer to wake-up time. Talk to your health care team about programming your pump to deliver more insulin near dawn.

6

Blood Glucose: Goals and Monitoring

People who don't have diabetes don't develop diabetic complications. Some people who have diabetes do develop complications: heart, kidney, eye, and nerve problems. The biggest difference between the two groups? Blood glucose levels. We now know from many studies that the closer your blood glucose levels are to the normal, nondiabetic range the lower your risk of developing diabetic complications.

Keeping your blood glucose levels close to normal ranges is often called "tight control." Tight control is not without some risk. The closer your blood glucose levels are to the normal range, the closer you are to hypoglycemia. You have to weigh the risks and benefits.

The suggested goals for most healthy, nonpregnant adults are in Table 6-1.

Children, older adults, and people with health problems may have higher goals. Women who are trying to conceive or are pregnant have lower goals.

If you aren't reaching goals that you and your health care provider think are reasonable, what can you do? Your doctor may want to refer you to an endocrinologist. If you're seeing only a doctor, try the team approach: work with a diabetes educator and/or dietitian in addition to your doctor. You may need a different insulin plan. For example, switching from two shots a day to three or more shots a day or an insulin pump will likely lead to better control.

When you feel frustrated, remember that diabetes is a complicated disease. Because everyone responds a little differently to diet, exercise, and insulin, the answers to how much to eat, how much to exercise, and how much insulin to take are not always obvious. You may find a support group helpful in reaching your goals.

Blood Glucose Monitoring Schedule

How often should you check your blood glucose level? Because you're the one who has to do it, only you can answer this question. Your doctor or diabetes educator can recommend a schedule, but it's really up to you: how often you're willing to do it, and what supplies you can afford. If you're trying for near-normal blood glucose levels, you'll be monitoring at least three or four times a day (Table 6-2).

Table 6-1. Blood Glucose Goals (mg/dl)

If Your Meter Gives Plasma Readings (Most newer meters do.)

	Normal (nondiabetic)	Goal	Additional action suggested if:
Before meals	less than 110	90–130	less than 90 or more than 150
At bedtime	less than 120	110–150	less than 110 or more than 180

If Your Meter Gives Whole Blood Readings

	Normal (nondiabetic)	Goal	Additional action suggested if:
Before meals	less than 100	80–120	less than 80 or more than 140
At bedtime	less than 110	100–140	less than 100 or more than 160

Check your blood glucose more often than usual when:

- you change your insulin injection plan, your meal plan, or your exercise routine.
- you are sick.
- you are pregnant or considering becoming pregnant.
- you have trouble recognizing the warning signals of hypoglycemia.
- your blood glucose levels have been dangerously high or low (outside your acceptable range).
- you start taking a medication that may affect blood glucose levels or your ability to recognize the warning signs of low blood glucose (ask your pharmacist about each prescription).

If you stop checking your blood sugar for a long period, ask yourself whether you're frustrated and trying to avoid facing problems in managing your diabetes. Monitoring can sometimes be depressing. You may get results that are way too high for no apparent reason. The best thing to do is to talk with your doctor or nurse educator. They can help you track down the culprit. Perhaps you need a new approach to insulin therapy. Don't give up on blood glucose monitoring.

Your Results

When you're learning how to do blood sugar monitoring, your first concern is doing it correctly. You may want to ask your doctor or nurse educator to watch you to check your method. If an unexpected reading shows up,

Table 6-2. Useful Times for Blood Glucose Checks

When	Why
Before meals	You can use these results to adjust your insulin dose using your sliding scale and pattern management.
One to two hours after a meal	To see the effects of various foods. To see whether your dose of rapid-acting insulin before the meal covered the meal.
Before bed	If it's low, you can eat a snack to prevent nighttime hypoglycemia. If it's low two nights in a row, you can lower the dose of insulin that is active at that time to prevent this.
When you feel that your blood glucose might be too low	Are you sweating because of your workout? Or are you having a low blood glucose reaction? A blood glucose check will tell you for sure. Without the results, you may tend to eat because you fear your blood glucose level is low. If it wasn't really low, it will go too high.
In the early morning, overnight.	Consider doing once a week or so, to see if you around 2 a.m. or 3 a.m. have low blood glucose reactions.
Before you drive or do work where a low glucose reaction will be dangerous	If it's low (70 mg/dl or less), treat it. Check again 15 minutes later to be sure your blood glucose is rising and that you are safe to drive or operate machinery. If not, treat again wait and till your blood glucose is normal. Always take along a snack in case the level drops later on.

check your technique and check whether the meter has a problem. Always keep your meter calibrated according to the manufacturer's instructions. When you get a new meter, learn how to take care of it and use it.

If you're faced with an unexpected high or low blood glucose reading and the meter is working fine, it's tempting to blame yourself. Maybe you know why your blood glucose is higher than you would like—the extra helping at dinner or failing to make it to your exercise class. Record your blood glucose honestly and be glad you can figure out why it's the level it is so the next time you can make an adjustment.

Writing down your daily results in a record book helps you know your blood glucose patterns. Ask your doctor or nurse educator for a record book with an easy-to-use format, or make your own. Some blood glucose meters store 10, 20, or as many as 250 test results in their memory, saving you from having to write your results down each time, but you still need to see the patterns. Share your records with each member of your health care team when you see them.

Your Blood Glucose Batting Average: A1C

If you checked your blood glucose level only in the morning, you might conclude that on average your blood glucose level runs about 90 mg/dl.

But you know that your blood glucose levels are higher after meals. If you checked

Not Enough or Too Much?

Ben Goldstein tested his blood glucose twice a day: before breakfast and before supper. His before-breakfast readings were fine: between 80 and 150 mg/dl. But his before-supper readings were high: 250 to 300 mg/dl.

Mr. Goldstein reported these results to his diabetes educator. "I must not have enough insulin in my blood then," he said. "Maybe I should be taking a bigger dose of long-acting insulin in the morning."

The diabetes educator looked at Mr. Goldstein's blood glucose log. She saw that he usually ate a large snack at 2:30 p.m. "I'm always really hungry then," he said.

The diabetes educator told Mr. Goldstein to check his blood glucose before his snack. When he did this, he was surprised to find that his glucose level was low. He then realized that his extreme hunger was a symptom of low blood glucose. He'd eat a big snack and then his blood glucose would be too high before supper.

The solution was to lower his morning dose of long-acting insulin.

your blood glucose more often and averaged all the numbers, you'd get a more accurate picture of what your average is.

The hemoglobin A1C test (A-one-C) is like having one hundred glucose checks every day. Here's how it works:

STATISTICS

In the DCCT, tight blood glucose control decreased the risk of developing neuropathy by:

- 69% among those who had no evidence of existing vascular complications at the start of the study

- 54% among those with mild or moderate vascular complications.

In an analysis of HMO utilization data in the state of Washington, a reduction of A1C of at least 1% resulted in a difference in health care costs of $685–$950 per person per year.

There's always some glucose in your blood. The same is true of people who don't have diabetes.

Glucose links up with the hemoglobin in your red blood cells. It "sugar coats" them. If you have a lot of glucose in your blood, more of your hemoglobin will have glucose attached. Once the glucose is attached, it's there for the life of that red blood cell—at most, about 120 days.

The percentage of your hemoglobin that has glucose attached can be measured with a blood test done by a lab. In a person who doesn't have diabetes, about 5% of the hemoglobin is "glycated" (has glucose attached). In people who have diabetes, the percentage is higher. How much higher depends on blood glucose levels. An A1C test shows you your average blood glucose level over the previous 2 to 3 months. Some people call it your blood glucose batting average.

A1C	Average Plasma* Glucose Level (mg/dl)
5	100
6	135
7	170
8	205
9	240
10	275
11	310
12	345

* Most meters give plasma readings.

(If your lab does a different type of glycated hemoglobin test, the percentages/plasma glucose values will be different from those above.)

What's the Goal?

The Diabetes Control and Complications Trial (DCCT) was a 10-year study of 1,441 people with type 1 diabetes. It compared two groups of people:

■ those on two-shot-a-day regimens who had an average A1C of about 9%
■ those on flexible insulin plans who had achieved an average A1C of just over 7%

The people in the second group worked hard to get their A1C's down. They used three or more shots a day or insulin pumps. They checked their blood glucose levels four or more times a day. They used sliding scales and pattern management (see chapter 5. Many used carbohydrate counting

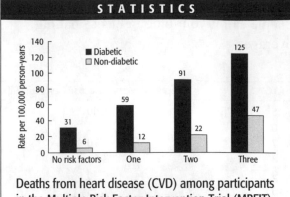

STATISTICS

Deaths from heart disease (CVD) among participants in the Multiple Risk Factor Intervention Trial (MRFIT), by diabetes status and number of CVD risk factors. Risk factors include total cholesterol >200 mg/dl, cigarette smoking, and hypertension.

Source: Data from Stamler et al.: Diabetes, other risk factors, and 12-year cardiovascular mortality for men screened in the Multiple Risk Factor Intervention Trial. *Diabetes Care* 2:434–444, 1993.

(see p. 83). (see p. 83) They worked with diabetes care teams that included dietitians, diabetes educators, endocrinologists, and mental health professionals.

People in the second group developed fewer diabetic complications (diabetic eye, kidney, and nerve disease) than those in the first group. Some people had complications at the start of the study. These complications slowed down in the second group. Overall, those in the second group had a reduction in risk of complications of about 60%.

Ask your health care team what your A1C goal is. Any reduction in A1C means a lower risk of complications. If your A1C is 9% and you get it down to 8%, you've reduced your risk of complications.

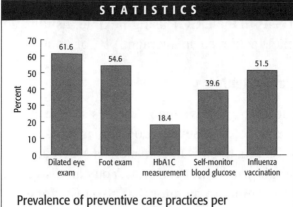

STATISTICS

**Prevalence of preventive care practices per
100 adults with diabetes, 41 U.S. states, 1997.**

Source: Data from Centers for Disease Control and Prevention. *Diabetes Surveillance,
1999.* Chapter 10: Preventive Care Practices. Division of Diabetes Translation, Centers for
Disease Control and Prevention, Atlanta, GA.

A reasonable goal for many adults is an A1C of less than 7%. An A1C of 6.5% without too many episodes of hypoglycemia per week is excellent control.

If your A1C is over 8%, work with your health care team. A change in your insulin plan or a new approach to matching food with insulin will likely get your A1C closer to normal levels.

If you are pregnant or trying to become pregnant, an A1C closer to 6% is recommended, as long as you're not having too many episodes of hypoglycemia.

Children under age 7, older adults, and people with certain health problems may have A1C goals higher than 7%. Hypoglycemia is particularly dangerous for them, and a higher A1C goal gives a bigger safety margin.

The teen years are a difficult time in many areas, including diabetes management.

An A1C goal of 7% might not be realistic. Teens in the DCCT using flexible insulin plans achieved an average A1C of about 8%.

How Often?

Most people have their A1C tests done at their doctor's. Several companies market A1C kits to consumers, such as Metrika's single-use home A1C test. You can also get a blood glucose monitor that also tests for a glycated protein, which tells you your average blood glucose level over the previous 2 weeks. The following chart suggests how often to have an A1C test.

If	Have A1C tests:
Your glucose control is stable and you're satisfied with it	Every 6 months
Your treatment plan has changed or you're not meeting your goals	Every 3 months
You're pregnant or trying to conceive	Every 4 to 6 weeks

THE LECTURE

As I backed out of my driveway, I felt like a rebellious teenager being forced to do something against my will. I tried to come up with a good excuse not to keep my doctor's appointment, but my responsible adult self won. "Just get it over with," I thought. "You know what they're going to tell you."

As I walked into the office, the smiling receptionist took my name and reached for my blood glucose monitor to make a computer printout. I did a tug of war with her in my mind, trying to decide if it was any of her business. The nurse weighed me, took my blood pressure, then stuck my finger for the inevitable glucose reading. "My, we're a little high today," she said frowning.

I moved to the examining room and listened to the discussions going on around me. Across the hall, there was an elderly man with a patch on his eye. He was holding the hand of his plump wife, their eyes riveted toward the door, listening for the doctor's footsteps. A baby was wailing in the next room, comforted by a mother with another 2-year-old attached to her leg.

An intern came in to do my work-up, and I remembered I wasn't in the mood for this. He sat down and began asking me questions. "Any headaches, stomachaches, muscle aches, history of heart disease, undue stress?"

I laughed and said, "Just check yes on everything. I'm sure it will happen sooner or later." He glanced at me then quickly continued. I answered with snappy replies, taking pleasure in making him nervous.

After he left, I sat resigned to my coming lecture and examined the computer printout from my meter. "It looks like you're a little high quite often, not just today," I said out loud, mimicking the nurse. But I could feel my rebellion giving way to the old familiar feeling of guilt for not taking control.

I know how to keep my blood sugar in control, but through the years I've found ways to rationalize a certain lack of control. When my children were young, I was afraid of having a hypoglycemic reaction. In a grocery store one day, I had to set my screaming baby in the cart while shocked onlookers watched me drink a can of orange juice right off the shelf. It was an experience I did not want to repeat, and I was willing to let my blood sugar go up a little to avoid it.

Even when my children were older, I still had to deal with a busy schedule, and I didn't want it interrupted by blood tests and shots. I didn't want to be in church or at a meeting that ran longer than expected and have to open a packet of crackers and munch on them while everyone stared.

I often wondered how many people with diabetes actually got a normal A1C blood test. I felt certain that those who did led lives that were completely controlled and inhibited by their disease.

I sat with my head in my hands and tried to come up with more reasons to justify my poor control. There weren't many left. The years of excuses were being replaced by the reality of changes in my vision and some unusual aches and pains.

I listened again to the young mother across the hall laughing with her children, and I knew she also had to juggle them, her home, and her control. I watched the older couple talking softly, worried about his complications and wishing for another chance. Who was I kidding? I had been rationalizing for years and soon it would be too late to turn back the clock. It was taking more energy now to fight the guilt than to fight the disease.

I was still deep in thought when the doctor came in. "Okay, dear," she said, "We're going to have to get tough on you."

"I know," I said, "I've got to keep to my diet plan, cut down on fats, and make sure I exercise three to four times a week."

"Very good," she said. "But most of all, I want you to get rid of the stress in your life. Learn how to take it easy on yourself."

Take it easy? This was not the lecture I had expected. My anger slipped away. As we talked, I began to realize that to really get rid of my stress, to "take it easy on myself," I had to give up those old companions, fear and guilt. Fear had bred the excuses that kept me from dealing with my diabetes, and the guilt that always followed became an overwhelming burden.

Nothing earth-shattering happened to me that day in the doctor's office, but I left with a renewed sense of purpose. For years, I had convinced myself that controlling my diabetes would be a burden. Yet by avoiding that responsibility, I was forced to bear a weighty load of guilt and self-doubt. Keeping my blood sugar in control will be a tough fight, but in the long run, I'm better off fighting diabetes than fighting myself.

JoAnn Westwood
Diabetes Forecast
1995

7

Tools of the Trade

Diabetes management involves both art and science. The art consists of lifestyle skills—diet, exercise, and stress management. Science includes a diabetes toolbox. It consists of everything from the simple finger-stick device for blood drop samples to the latest blood glucose data management system.

The best catalog for a diabetes toolbox is the American Diabetes Association *Resource Guide*, published every January in *Diabetes Forecast* magazine and as a separate supplement (see p. 189). This guide lists and describes all available diabetes care tools on the market.

Blood Glucose Meters

Your blood glucose meter (or monitor) is your diabetes intelligence service. It warns you of blood glucose levels out of your range so you can take action.

Most states require that insurance cover meters and strips. If your insurance offers meters and strips through a mail-order or prescription benefit program, you'll need to get a physician's prescription to be reimbursed.

If you don't have insurance, you can almost always find a deal on a meter with rebates and special purchase offers. Check with your diabetes educator or pharmacist and keep an eye on ads. Check the *Diabetes Forecast Resource Guide*. You'll probably find a bargain, especially in shopping for strips.

Medicare covers glucose meters, test strips, and lancets. For information about Medicare's coverage of diabetes supplies, contact:

The Center for Medicare and Medicaid
    Services (CMS)
7500 Security Blvd.
Baltimore, MD 21244
1-800-MEDICARE (1-800-633-4227)
    (English and Spanish)
TTY/TDD 1-877-486-2048
via the internet www.medicare.gov

The 2002 *Resource Guide* listed more than 30 models of blood glucose meter systems. All perform the basic job of reporting glucose levels in your blood. Some models, however, make more sense for you than others. To choose the right meter, consider:

▓ **Sample site and size.** Meters that need smaller-sized blood drops may be easier for those with poor circulation in their hands or who must test in cold environments. Some meters allow you to take samples from the forearm or thigh rather than the fingertip.

▓ **Meter size.** Smaller meters slip easily into a shirt pocket when you're on the move. On the other hand, they get lost easily in a deep, dark handbag. The larger-sized meters stick out in both situations.

▓ **Your dexterity.** If you have trouble with small hand and finger movements, ask your diabetes educator or pharmacist to let you try the recommended meter before you buy it. Try meters that require less handling or use larger strips. You may also find it easier to use a meter that has strips that come in a vial, rather than individually wrapped in foil. The foil wrappings can be quite hard to remove.

▓ **Test timing.** How long are you willing to wait? Some meters take a minute to give results. Some take as little as 5 seconds. These ultra-fast machines are especially useful in work and social situations, where it feels as if an extra 30 seconds really does make a difference.

▓ **Your vision.** If you have any trouble seeing or have some degree of color blindness, be sure that you have no trouble reading the digital display. If you have severe vision loss, make sure that a close companion or family member is trained in the use of your meter and the rest of the diabetes toolbox so they can help you when necessary. For some meters, you can buy a voice synthesizer accessory that "talks" (in English or another language) you through the procedure and results.

■ **Support system.** If you are using a meter for the first time, consider one that offers a video that teaches you how to test. Make sure the company has a 24-hour 800 number to call when you have problems with the meter. Also check that your health care professional is familiar with the model you buy.

■ **Ease of upkeep.** Each batch of testing strips is slightly different from the last. When you open a new batch, the meter must be calibrated to account for these differences. Then you will get accurate readings despite tiny differences in strips. Some machines calibrate completely by themselves. You don't have to do anything with a new batch of strips. On some models, however, the calibration procedures can be a little tedious. Some have a two-step procedure using a special strip. Instructions are usually included in every package of strips, so don't panic if you've lost your meter instruction manual.

■ **Meter memory.** If you have trouble keeping a written log book, select a meter that stores your results in memory. At night you can record the day's readings in your logbook or computer.

Your health care team may prefer you use a certain brand of meter that allows them to connect your meter to their computer and download your readings. Ask your diabetes educator or team member if they do.

If you're comfortable using computers, you can buy software for downloading your results. Each brand of meter has specific software. If you're interested, contact the meter manufacturer. They'll tell you how to get it and what it costs. Insurance plans don't cover software or cables.

■ **Language.** Some meter systems can display in English, Spanish, or up to seven other languages.

■ **Battery and machine replacement.** Just like flashlights and TV remote controls, meters need batteries. Each model handles batteries differently. A few have permanent batteries, which usually last for a few years. Then you have to replace the meter. For most meters, the batteries are standard electronic-equipment batteries. You buy the replacements and insert them yourself. Depending on how often you test, batteries can last months to years. It's always best to have one on hand before you need it.

■ **Your insurance coverage.** Your insurance program or company health plan may want you to use a specific meter. Check this out before you buy and also find out if you're covered for the strips.

■ **Your need/desire for other test results.** A few blood glucose meters also test for lipids, ketones, and glycated proteins.

These features are usually not needed unless your doctor suggests you need to do these tests at home.

No Matter Which Meter You Choose . . .

When you buy your meter, be sure it has been set to the correct date and time. Ask your pharmacist or diabetes educator to show you how.

Meters and strips sometimes malfunction and give false results. This can have important health consequences. For instance, an elderly man with diabetes started having low meter results without any symptoms. His doctor lowered his insulin dose. Fortunately, the man attended a diabetes education program just after this change. The educators at the program discovered that his meter was showing incorrect results. It turns out he had left his strips in a hot car. He bought new strips and brought his blood glucose levels down using his original insulin dose.

▓ **Test your machine and strips for accuracy** using a standard control solution. These solutions have a known concentration of glucose that you compare to your meter's result. Do this monthly or according to manufacturer's instructions, and also when you suspect your meter is not working correctly.

▓ **Take your meter with you** for diabetes appointments. Take a meter reading within a few minutes of having blood drawn for laboratory glucose tests. Compare the results. If your meter is off by more than 15%, call the manufacturer for possible replacement.

Finger-Sticking Devices and Lancets

Meters always come with a lancet device. The devices often have adjustments for how deep the lancets poke into your finger or they have separate caps that control depth. Use the shallowest poke possible to draw blood. If your device comes without an adjustment or it hurts too much for you, talk to your diabetes educator about finding a device that's right for you.

Some people use lancets without the lancing device to sample their blood. This takes some practice and usually hurts more.

If you have dexterity limitations, look for an automatic lancing device that resets easily with a simple push-pull movement.

Record-Keeping

The logbook? This low-tech equipment is often overlooked as an important piece of the diabetes toolbox. Everybody gets one free with their first meter. After that, they can be surprisingly hard to find. Pharmacies may or may not carry them. If you have trouble finding them, ask your diabetes educator for some or where you can find them. You can also call the toll-free number for your meter company and ask for more.

If you have complications of diabetes or other medical conditions, you might want to use a spiral-bound notebook instead. You can list a variety of symptoms or situations

relevant to your medical condition. Note-
books also offer lots of room to write for
people whose fingers might be a little stiff.

Data-management systems automatically
record various aspects of your diabetes control each time you perform a blood glucose
test. These systems can store hundreds of test
results and other information (depending on
the system), such as time, date, insulin type
and dose, and exercise. Some meters have
built-in data-management systems; other systems must be connected to the meter.

If your doctor or diabetes educator has a
personal computer that's compatible with
your system, he or she can get a complete
and accurate record of your test results over a
period of time. Some systems allow downloading to your doctor's computer by
modem.

After downloading, the information can
be plotted on a graph. You and your health
care team can see patterns in your blood glucose levels.

Before you buy, check:

■ **Compatibility.** Make sure the system can
  "talk" to your computer and your doctor's
  computer.
■ **Ease of use.** If you can, try several before
  buying. Ask your diabetes educator to
  recommend one.
■ **Expense.** These systems are a luxury, not
  a necessity. You can see blood glucose
  patterns with a detailed handwritten logbook or with simple downloading software discussed earlier.

Odds-n-Ends

People with diabetes should round out their tool kit with a few other items. One is the carrying case for diabetes supplies. Have you ever tried to stuff your meter, syringes, insulin, alcohol wipes, and so forth into a purse or briefcase? If you have, you'll know why you need a special carrying bag. These cases do two things for you. First, they organize all your supplies. Second, they insulate your insulin from hot or cold temperatures. They also separate your diabetes supplies from other baggage—avoiding the beginner's nightmare of having supplies lost in a suitcase gone astray at the airport.

Where to Buy

Some pharmacies specialize in diabetes supplies, carrying a large number of brands of meters and other supplies. In addition to medical supplies, you may find low-calorie foods, candies, books, and information on local diabetes events and organizations.

Diabetes supply specialty stores offer another shopping option. To find one, call your local ADA chapter, or check in the phone book under "Medical Supplies" or "Diabetes." If you're lucky enough to have one in the neighborhood, you may be able to one-stop-shop for many nonprescription items. In diabetes shops, you can actually compare models, ask questions, and receive training on complicated tools.

You might choose to use mail-order. Timing is critical. Be sure to order your

strips, insulin, and other equipment at least
2 weeks in advance. Waiting until the last
moment will leave you high and dry for medication and test supplies. Also, if you are
insured, starting up with a mail-order house
takes additional time up front. They must
confirm your insurance coverage before filling your first order.

8

Food

You're eating healthy. Or you're eating all-American meals. Or you're living on caffeine and junk food. No matter what you eat, you want to reach your blood glucose goals.

When you know how different foods affect your blood glucose levels, you can make decisions about when, what, and how much to eat. That helps you reach your blood glucose goals.

The Big Three

Meals are made up of various amounts of

- carbohydrate (starches and sugar)
- fat
- protein

These three nutrients give us calories (a measurement of food energy).

Little of the fat and protein you eat turns up as glucose. The carbohydrate you eat is broken down into glucose (your body's preferred source of energy), which then moves into your bloodstream. This begins happening within minutes after you eat and continues for several hours.

By matching the insulin you take to the carbohydrate you eat, you can improve your blood glucose control.

Diabetes Food Pyramid

The first step in diabetes meal planning is to know the content of the foods you eat. Since carbohydrates have a direct effect on blood glucose, you'll want to know which foods contain a lot of carbohydrate and which do not.

You're probably familiar with the USDA Food Guide Pyramid. It's on many food packages. (Check your crackers or bread.)

The American Diabetes Association and The American Dietetic Association adapted the Food Guide Pyramid for people with diabetes (p. 79). A few foods were shifted into different sections based on how they affect blood glucose levels. Starchy vegetables—potatoes, corn, peas—were moved to the bottom layer, with the grains. Those vegetables raise blood glucose more than, say, spinach, given equal portion sizes. Beans have protein, but they also have carbohydrate, unlike other protein foods such as fish and eggs. So beans were moved to the section with grains as well.

Diabetes Food Pyramid

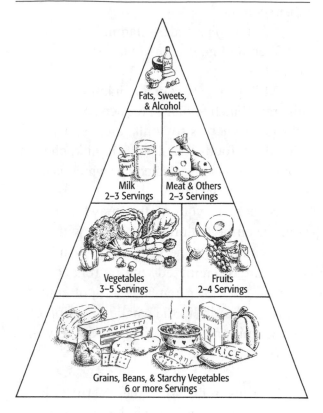

Foods with carbohydrate are:

- Grains, Beans, and Starchy Vegetables
- Fruits
- Milk Products
- Sweets

Are the carbohydrates different in these different sections? Yes and no.

Yes. In terms of overall health, some sections are better than others. Whole grains, beans, and starchy vegetables provide vitamins, minerals, and fiber. Notice that their section is the biggest, meaning healthy meals have more servings from this section than from the other sections.

Fruit also provides vitamins, minerals, and fiber, and no saturated fat nor cholesterol.

Milk products contain vitamins and minerals. Fat-free dairy products, or milk substitutes such as soy milk, are healthy. But other dairy foods (whole or 2% milk, cheese, sour cream) have saturated fat, which is not good for your heart.

Sweets, as your mother may have told you, are empty calories—calories with little if any vitamins, minerals, or fiber. And sweets are often mixed with fat (chocolate, pastries), so they often have a *lot* of empty calories. They're in the smallest section of the pyramid; a healthy diet has few servings of sweets.

No. In terms of the effect these carbohydrate foods have on your blood glucose levels, no, they are not different from each other. Two hours after a meal, a serving (1/2 cup) of mashed potatoes will have raised your blood glucose about as much as a serving (1/2 cup) of ice cream.

"What?! Is Sugar OK?"

Despite bad press, sugar really isn't off-limits to people with diabetes. Sugars are carbohydrates. In terms of blood glucose control, there is no evidence that people with diabetes should avoid sugars in favor of other foods that also contain carbohydrate.

How much you eat, how quickly you eat, the way the food has been prepared, and the combination of foods eaten are what determine how quickly food is digested and absorbed. For example, eating foods containing fat slows down their absorption.

So, your first priority should be to think about your carbohydrate intake and how it changes your blood glucose level. If you aim to eat a certain number of carbohydrates each day, and you eat a lot of sugary foods, you'll get to eat only a few of the more nutrient-rich starchy foods.

"But Sugar Is 'Fast,' Right?"

Well . . . yes and no. We know—you've heard it a hundred times: If you're having a low blood glucose reaction, eat or drink a "fast-acting" carbohydrate. Fruit juice or anything with sugar are often given as examples.

But actually, if you happen to be sitting in front of a glass of milk when you're beginning to go low, it would be fine to drink. A cup has about 15 grams of carbohydrate in the form of a natural sugar. Your digestive system breaks it down quickly, and the glucose is absorbed. Sucrose (table sugar) actually requires more processing by the body to turn it all into glucose. For more on treating "lows," see pp. 96–99.

Balance

Carbohydrate raises blood glucose; insulin lowers it. How do you balance the two?

■ **If you're on a structured insulin plan**, you have the same amount of insulin active at the same times each day. So you need to eat about the same amount of carbohydrate at a given meal to keep your blood glucose levels more predictable.

■ **If you take aspart, lispro, or regular** insulin before meals, you can decide how much carbohydrate you're going to eat (or even whether to eat at all) and then take the amount of insulin that will cover the meal.

There are several meal planning tools you can use to balance carbohydrate and insulin.

Exchange Lists for Meal Planning

In *Exchange Lists for Meal Planning,* by the American Diabetes Association and The American Dietetic Association, foods are split into three large groups:

■ Carbohydrate
■ Meat and meat substitutes
■ Fat

Carbohydrate has subgroups:

■ Starch (breads, crackers, cereals, starchy vegetables, pasta)
■ Fruit (fresh, canned, juice)
■ Milk
■ Other carbohydrates (sugars, sweets, desserts)
■ Vegetables

The "exchange lists" are lists of food and their serving sizes. Each "exchange" has about the same amount of carbohydrate, fat, and protein as every other food on that list. Any food on a list can be exchanged for any other food on the same list.

A dietitian can work up an exchange meal plan for you. Your meal plan might call for:

- Breakfast: 2 starch, 1 fruit, and 1 milk
- Lunch: 2 starch, 2 vegetable, 2 fruit, 2 meat
- Supper: 3 starch, 2 vegetable, 1 fruit, 1 milk, 1 meat

One day breakfast can be oatmeal with raisins and a glass of milk. Another day it can be cold cereal with milk plus yogurt and fruit. As long as you stick to the general template of 2 starch, 1 fruit, and 1 milk, you'll get about the same amount of carbohydrate at each breakfast. That's good for blood glucose control.

When you follow your exchange plan throughout the day, you get a balanced diet with foods from different food groups. That's good for overall health.

Carbohydrate Counting

A popular meal-planning tool is carbohydrate counting. Use carb counting if you want:

- consistency in your carbohydrate intake, or
- the flexibility to change meal size and insulin dose.

We'll start with consistency, and we'll use the exchange lists as a starting point. The breakfast in the exchange section above calls for 2 starch, 1 fruit, and 1 milk. One starch exchange has about 15 grams of carbohydrate. So does one fruit exchange. One milk exchange has about 12 grams of carbohydrate—about the same. So what's to stop you from eating 3 starches and 1 milk for breakfast? Or 4 starches? You can do that, and your blood glucose will rise about the same amount.

A "carbohydrate choice" is a serving of food that contains about 15 grams of carbohydrate; 1 starch, 1 milk, 1 fruit, or 1 "other carbohydrate" exchange is 1 carb choice. In carb-counting language, the breakfast above is 4 carb choices.

A vegetable exchange has only 5 grams of carbohydrate. You don't count nonstarchy vegetables unless you eat a lot at one sitting.

You can expand your choice of foods beyond what's in the exchange lists. Look on the Nutrition Facts of any packaged food. You'll find how much carbohydrate is in a serving. You want to pay attention to Total Carbohydrate. You can ignore the line for Sugars. Sugars are included in Total Carbohydrate.

Note that a food label serving size is often—but not always—the same as an exchange list serving size.

	Exchange Serving Size	Food Label Serving Size
Fruit juice	1/2 cup (4 oz)	1 cup (8 oz)

Raspberry Juice Drink

Nutrition Facts
Serving Size 8 fl oz
Servings Per Container 2

Amount Per Serving	
Calories 110	Calories from Fat 0

Total Fat 0g	
Saturated Fat 0g	
Cholesterol 0mg	
Sodium 5mg	
Total Carbohydrate 27g	
Dietary Fiber 1g	
Sugars 25g	
Protein 1g	

One serving of Raspberry Juice Drink (above) has 27 grams of carbohydrate. That's about 2 carb choices. Note that if you drink the entire container—easy to do!—you will have drunk 54 grams of carbohydrate, or about 3 1/2 carb choices.

Advanced Carbohydrate Counting

During the week, a cup of black coffee with no sugar at 7 a.m. is your entire breakfast. But on the weekends, you get up later and have pancakes with syrup and a glass of orange juice.

Coffee has no carbohydrate. A stack of pancakes and all the trimmings has a lot.

Can you do that? Yes—if you use rapid- or short-acting insulin before meals and know how to adjust your dose for the size of the meal.

On weekdays, you'd check your blood glucose level in the morning. If it's in your target range, you'd take no rapid- or short-acting insulin, because there's no carbohydrate to cover. You'd still take your long-acting insulin.

(If your blood glucose was out of your goal range, you'd correct for that. You might take a little insulin to correct a high, using a sliding scale you and your health care team have worked out, or eat a snack to correct a low. If you're low or high several times in a row, it's time for some pattern management (see chapter 5).

On weekends, you'd take a mealtime dose of rapid- or short-acting insulin before the pancake breakfast.

How much insulin would you take? You'd count the grams of carbohydrate you're going to eat and dose accordingly.

People with type 1 diabetes typically need 1 unit of rapid- or short-acting insulin to cover 10 to 15 grams of carbohydrate. It depends on how sensitive to insulin you are. A 1:15 insulin-to-carbohydrate ratio works for many adults. People with little body fat are usually more sensitive to insulin, and a unit of insulin will cover more carbohydrate for them. The higher the second number, the more insulin-sensitive the person is, and the less insulin he or she needs to cover a given amount of carbohydrate.

Young children are usually very sensitive to insulin; adolescents are not. A child might use a ratio of 1 unit for 20 to 25 grams of carbohydrate; an adolescent might use a

1:10 ratio. In other words, to cover a meal containing 50 grams of carbohydrate, a young child may need only 2 units of rapid-acting insulin, but a teen might need 5 units.

You don't have to figure this out on your own! Your dietitian or diabetes educator will look at your total insulin dose and your blood glucose records, do some calculations, and estimate your ratio. Blood glucose monitoring before and after meals will let you know if you need to change the ratio.

You might change the ratio several times over the course of several months before you hit on the best ratio. And you might have different ratios at different times of the day, because your insulin sensitivity changes during the day. You might have a different ratio on days that you exercise, because exercise makes you more sensitive to insulin—1 unit will cover more carbohydrate.

Sound kind of complicated? It is. Get guidance from your dietitian and diabetes educator throughout the learning process. You won't always be measuring, weighing, and scribbling on paper. It will soon become second nature—and you'll love the flexibility and the feeling of control it gives you.

See p. 166 for more information on how to find a dietitian and p. 202 for a record-keeping form.

Let Him Eat Cake

Jordan was newly diagnosed with diabetes. He was prescribed set doses of insulin twice a day.

His mother had to absorb a lot of information in a short time. She remembered that his meals needed to be consistent, so she served Jordan the same kind of sandwich every day for lunch. She also thought that sugar was off limits, so she wasn't allowing Jordan to eat his favorite cereal for breakfast, and she had told Jordan he couldn't have cake on his upcoming birthday.

A week after Jordan's release from the hospital, a dietitian/diabetes educator made a home visit. Jordan and his mother learned that the carbohydrate content of his meals needed to be consistent, but that this could be done with different foods. Jordan could eat spaghetti one day, cold cereal another day, and a sandwich the third day, as long as all those lunches had about the same amount of carbohydrate.

Jordan's mother learned to look at the "Total Carbohydrate" line of the Nutrition Facts, not the "Sugars" line. She saw that Jordan's favorite cereal had about the same amount of Total Carbohydrate as the less-sugary cereal that she had been allowing. But now that she was looking at food labels, she saw that her cereal was made with whole grains and had more fiber. She and Jordan reached a compromise: He would mix the cereals.

Jordan's mother also learned how to work cake into Jordan's meal plan for his birthday.

Sugar Smackeroos

Nutrition Facts

Serving Size 1 cup (30g)

Amount Per Serving (without milk)

Calories 120   Calories from Fat 10

Total Fat 1g

  Saturated Fat 0g

Cholesterol 0mg

Sodium 210mg

Total Carbohydrate 25g

  Dietary Fiber 1g

  Sugars 13g

  Other Carbohydrate 11g

Protein 2g

Oat Circles

Nutrition Facts

Serving Size 1 cup

Amount Per Serving (without milk)

Calories 130   Calories from Fat 0

Total Fat 2g

  Saturated Fat 0g

Cholesterol 0mg

Sodium 280mg

Total Carbohydrate 22g

  Dietary Fiber 3g

  Sugars 1g

  Other Carbohydrate 18g

Protein 3g

Lows and Highs

Hypoglycemia

A blood glucose level that is too low is called hypoglycemia. (Compare this with *hyper-glycemia*, an abnormally high blood glucose level.) Ask your doctor what blood glucose levels to watch out for. In general, if you're a healthy adult, below 70 mg/dl is considered too low. The "safe level" is higher in:

- **Children under age 7.** Hypoglycemia is rough on the developing brains of young children. In addition, young children often don't realize that they're going low, so they're likely to drop even lower.
- **People with heart problems**, because hypoglycemia causes a rapid heart beat.
- **Elderly people**, especially those living alone.
- **People in jobs** where hypoglycemia would be dangerous.

For people with type 1 diabetes, hypo-glycemia is a fact of life. On average, people with type 1 diabetes have one or two low blood glucose reactions a week.

"It's very hard to tell when you have low blood sugar and when you're just pumping adrenaline from the gig. The answer is to do a blood test."

—Ray Anderson, jazz trombonist

Many things can cause too much of a drop in blood glucose levels. They include too much insulin, too little food, a delayed meal, a meal with too little carbohydrate, excess exercise, or alcohol on an empty stomach. Hypoglycemia usually occurs just before meals, after strenuous exercise, and when insulin is peaking. Sometimes it occurs at night when you're sleeping.

Each person's reaction to low blood glucose brings out a different set of symptoms, and you won't have them all:

Symptoms of Mild Hypoglycemia

Shakiness, nervousness, sweating, irritability, impatience, chills and clamminess, rapid heartbeat, anxiety, light-headedness, and hunger.

Symptoms of Moderate and Severe Hypoglycemia

Sleepiness, anger, stubbornness, sadness, lack of coordination, blurred vision, nausea, tingling or numbness in the lips or tongue, headaches, strange behavior, delirium, confusion, personality change, and unconsciousness. These symptoms mean your brain is not getting enough glucose.

Symptoms of Nighttime Hypoglycemia

Certain signs are clues that you've had hypoglycemia during the night. Do you find your pajamas and sheets damp in the morning? Have you had restless sleep and nightmares? When you wake up, do you have a headache or still feel tired? Check your blood glucose levels around 2 a.m. or 3 a.m. for a couple of days to find out if you're going low at night. If you are, tell your health care team. They'll advise you on how to change your diabetes plan to prevent nighttime lows. (Also see p. 50.)

Symptoms in Children

Be alert to subtle clues from your child. For example, does the teacher report that your child does well in math class but doesn't pay attention during spelling? Does spelling come right before lunch? Maybe your child's blood glucose is low then. Arrange for your child's blood glucose to be checked at that time a couple of days in a row to see. If that's not possible, have your child eat a small snack (for example, a cup of skim milk) before spelling class and see if that helps.

Missing The Signs

You may not get or you might miss the early warning signs of hypoglycemia if:

▩ You have even mild autonomic neuropathy (nerve damage from diabetes).

▩ You have had diabetes for many years.

This seems to be linked to longer length of time with diabetes rather than diabetic autonomic neuropathy. Even people without autonomic neuropathy can have this problem. So blood glucose monitoring becomes even more important as your years with diabetes increase.

▩ You have had a recent bout of hypoglycemia.

Hypoglycemia makes your body less reactive to the next bout. You may not get symptoms until your blood glucose drops to even lower levels.

▩ You're keeping your blood glucose levels near the normal range.

Your body gets used to often being close to 70 mg/dl, and it doesn't react as much when you dip below that. That's why it's so important to monitor your blood glucose levels more when you aim for near-normal glucose levels.

Is It Really Low?

You can develop symptoms of hypoglycemia when your blood glucose is falling rapidly but is still above 70 mg/dl. For example, if your blood glucose drops from 180 to 100 mg/dl rapidly, you might get chills or start sweating.

Hypoglycemic symptoms are a clue but not the full story. You must ask yourself, "Do I really have low blood glucose right now?" The answer is found by checking your blood glucose. If you don't find out for sure whether you're low, you may be treating a "non-low" which leads to high glucose levels and possibly weight gain.

On the other hand, you might brush off symptoms. Early warning signs are easy to miss. Yes, your heart will beat faster if you're anxious about a test or a new job. But it could be hypoglycemia. Is your sadness due to a fight with a friend, or is it hypo-glycemia? Don't wait to see if the symptoms go away. Only a blood glucose check can tell you for sure.

What if you don't have your glucose monitor when you feel that your blood glu-cose is going low? Don't wait. When in doubt, always treat. A possible check is to take your pulse. Your heart beats faster with hypoglycemia. Of course, you will have to know what your normal resting heart rate is. If your heart rate is significantly high (for example, your resting heart rate is 76, but now it is over 100), you are likely having a reaction. If your heart rate does not come down after aerobic exercise, you might suspect hypoglycemia.

Over time, you'll gain confidence in your ability to manage your diabetes. You may think you can check your blood glucose less often. Be careful that you don't convince yourself that you can tell your glucose level by how you feel. Research shows that few people can guess their blood glucose level. Guessing is dangerous, particularly if your blood glucose level tends to fall with very little warning.

Treatment

When you're having a low blood glucose reaction, your body needs glucose fast. You need to eat or drink something with sugar or starch. By now, you probably have your favorite form of "pocket sugar" that you keep with you at all times.

When you first notice a reaction, do a blood test if at all possible. Then follow the 15/15 rule: Take about 15 grams of glucose or other carbohydrate (about 1 fruit or 1 starch exchange). Retest your blood after 15 minutes. If your blood glucose hasn't come up enough, take another 15 grams of carbohydrate and retest in 15 minutes. After you treat the reaction, if it's the middle of the night or if your next meal is more than an hour away, also eat a snack.

Symptoms of hypoglycemia often linger after blood glucose levels are back in the normal range. Resist the urge to eat until you feel better, or your blood glucose will likely go too high.

You find similar foods on every list of foods to treat a low. Each of these has about 15 grams of carbohydrate:

- half a can of regular soda
- 1/2 cup (4 oz) of orange juice
- 5 to 7 LifeSavers
- 10 gumdrops
- 2 large lumps of sugar
- 1 tablespoon of honey or corn syrup
- a tube of Cake Mate decorator gel
- 1 cup of skim milk
- 2 to 5 glucose tablets, depending on the brand.

For quick, certain relief, glucose tablets or gels (available at pharmacies) are best. These are already the simplest sugar, so the glucose reaches your blood more quickly. Most of the food or drinks listed above contain sucrose, which is glucose plus fructose. The body must process the fructose to turn it into glucose. Another point in their favor is that you probably won't be tempted to snack on them because tablets and gel seem more like medication. However, the commercial glucose products cost more than other foods containing sugar.

If your low blood glucose reaction has left you conscious but unable to chew, gels are a good choice. Someone may have to assist you by putting the gel inside your mouth between your cheek and gum.

Everyone has a favorite way of treating hypoglycemia, but do you really know its exact effect on you? Try this: When your blood glucose is about 100 mg/dl or less, take your favorite "low" treatment. Wait 15 minutes. Then retest your blood. How much did your blood glucose rise—25, 30, 50, or more? You now know how to gauge your response to your level of hypoglycemia. You won't be as likely to overtreat and shoot your blood glucose up too high. And you won't be as likely to overeat and gain weight.

Try this test with other choices. You may find that one food is faster and has more predictable results than another.

You don't want to treat a reaction by eating ice cream or chocolate. These contain a lot of fat, which slows the absorption of the sugar. They also have a lot of calories, which can lead to weight gain.

Your most important protection against hypoglycemia is checking your blood glucose levels. With this information, you can figure out how to balance food, activity, and insulin.

Severe Hypoglycemia

If the early signs and symptoms of hypoglycemia go unnoticed or unheeded, you could develop severe hypoglycemia. You get so drowsy or confused that even if someone hands you juice, you can't drink it. (If they try to force you to drink or eat, you could choke.) With severe hypoglycemia, you can go unconscious or have a convulsion.

Severe hypoglycemia is a real emergency. Someone needs to call 911 or give you a shot of glucagon.

Glucagon is a hormone that makes the liver release stored glucose. This raises the blood glucose level, and the person usually regains consciousness. Glucagon doesn't work in people who have no stores of glucose in the liver, such as alcoholics.

Glucagon is injected like insulin. Someone you trust needs to be trained in how to fill the special glucagon syringe and to inject you. (See p. 185.) Ask your family to go with you to a training session. Your doctor or nurse may show them how in a special office visit or they may suggest that all of you attend a class.

You should respond to glucagon in 2–10 minutes. When you are fully awake, you should be offered sips of juice. If you keep that down, you should be offered food.

If you are still confused or unconscious 15 minutes after the glucagon injection, someone should call 911.

After the crisis is over, notify your doctor that you had a low severe enough to need glucagon.

Anyone who uses insulin needs to have glucagon in the house. It's available by prescription. It stays good for two years after manufacture. When it expires, get a new glucagon kit. Then have someone in your family practice mixing up the glucagon in the expired kit.

Reducing Your Risk

Ask for help. Do you feel comfortable telling friends and a few colleagues at work, school, and even the gym about the possibility of your low blood glucose? During a hypoglycemic reaction, you can become so confused and irritable that you refuse help. Those around you may have to be persistent in the face of your denial. They can save you from a coma and a trip to the hospital by making sure you take some form of glucose quickly. Life is easier and safer if those with whom you spend the most time can spot a low blood glucose reaction and know what to do about it.

Teach your family and friends about treating hypoglycemia as they seem ready and able to learn. Remember how over- whelming the amount of information seemed to you at first. You don't have to teach them all by yourself. There are pamphlets and books. Perhaps your family would benefit from attending a class together.

"You know the first thing most people who are having an insulin reaction say? 'Oh, I'm fine. There's nothing at all wrong with me. I don't need anything.' "
   –Mark Collie, singer-songwriter, who depends on frequent blood glucose checks and his band members to let him know when he's going low

---

You may feel embarrassed by symp- toms that your hypoglycemia may cause. But being cranky and irritable at times is not too different from the way some of your friends act from time to time. And everyone can seem clumsy or confused once in awhile. Your friends and family will learn to be tolerant even when you're obnoxious and refuse help. You must be willing to let others know of the possibility of hypoglycemia and how to help.

Wear medical identification at all times. Hypoglycemia is sometimes mistaken for drunkenness. Medical IDs tell strangers and emergency workers that you are probably having an insulin reaction. You can get necklaces, bracelets, sneaker tags, and watch charms. Emergency workers will probably look for neck chains and bracelets first. Also carry medical ID in your wallet.

Don't take unnecessary chances. Although time alone is important for everyone, you need not take unnecessary chances. Why exercise late in the afternoon without taking a snack and checking your glucose levels? Why drive all day without stopping for lunch? Why swim alone? These are just a few examples of incidents where you can reduce the possibility of hypoglycemia. Be sensible. It's your life.

Remember that exercise lowers blood glucose. Hypoglycemia is common 4 to 10 hours after exercise. Monitor your blood glucose levels to find out how your body reacts. See chapter 10 for more information on exercise and hypoglycemia.

Adjust for sexual activity. Are you prone to hypoglycemia with exercise or during the night? If you have sex at night, when your blood glucose levels typically dip anyway, you may need to have a snack before or after sexual activity. Some people who wear insulin pumps take the pumps off during sex and don't miss the insulin at all.

Watch your alcohol intake. Your liver has two important jobs. When you're not eating (between meals and overnight), your liver releases glucose into your bloodstream. This gives you some protection from low blood glucose. Your liver also has the job of clearing toxins from your blood.

Alcohol is a toxin. When you drink alcohol, your liver gives priority to detoxifying your blood, and it doesn't release stored glucose. Therefore, alcohol increases the risk of hypoglycemia.

Alcohol can contribute to a low even 8 hours after your last drink. Physical activity when you're drinking, such as dancing, lowers blood glucose even more.

The standard advice is to drink only with meals. But this may not be enough to protect you from low blood glucose. Alcohol's blocking effect on the liver lasts much longer than the glucose from your meal.

If you drink during the day, check your blood glucose level every 2 hours for 8 hours. If it's low, eat a carbohydrate snack.

If you drink in the evening, keep track of the number of servings of alcohol you drink. Each of the following is one serving of alcohol: 12 oz of beer, 4 oz of wine, one shot of liquor.

Before you go to bed, eat 10–15 grams of carbohydrate for each serving of alcohol you drank. If you normally eat a bedtime snack, eat your usual snack plus the extra carbohydrate. Eat this snack even if your blood glucose level is within or above your goal range (100–140 mg/dl for most people).

Keep in mind that alcohol and extra snacks add calories to your diet. Also be aware that alcohol affects motivation. You may find that even one glass of wine with dinner makes you less interested in accomplishing anything else that evening from folding the laundry to monitoring your blood glucose levels.

Diabetic Ketoacidosis

We so often talk of insulin lowering blood glucose that it sounds as if that's its only job: to simply clear glucose from the bloodstream. But its real job is to move glucose into cells so the cells can use it for energy.

If you don't have enough insulin in your system, glucose can't get into your muscle cells. They're starved for a source of energy. So the body starts to break down some of its stored fat. A by-product of this breakdown of fat is ketones. Normally, the body gets rid of ketones in the urine. If they form faster than the body can get rid of them, ketones build up in your blood, and your blood turns acidic.

"I thought I could handle it myself."
—Patricia Johnson, who caught a mid-winter bug and then landed in the hospital for two days with diabetic ketoacidosis.

A lack of insulin also lets glucose build up in your blood. Your body tries to get rid of the excess glucose by producing more urine, and you get dehydrated.

A build-up of ketones plus dehydration equals diabetic ketoacidosis (DKA). DKA can cause breathing difficulties, coma, shock, pneumonia, and even death. Small children may experience swelling of the brain (cerebral edema).

DKA Can Develop When

■ **A bottle of your insulin goes bad.** If your insulin doesn't look normal or is past the expiration date, start a new bottle.

■ **You're using an insulin pump and the tubing gets blocked or the needle comes out and you don't know it.** Alarms should warn you if there's a clog in the tubing, but machines sometimes malfunction.

■ **A dose of insulin is skipped.** Psychological or social pressures may cause people to skip doses. Teenagers may not be ready to take responsibility for their own glucose checks and injections. People who are emotionally or mentally disturbed and people with eating disorders may drop their therapy.

■ **You take your normal dose of insulin but it's not enough.** When the body has to deal with an infection, a sickness such as the flu, or a stressful situation, hormones cause the liver to release stored glucose. These hormones also make your muscles somewhat resistant to insulin, so blood glucose doesn't enter the tissues. Fatty acids are used as an energy source instead, and ketones form.

If you're sick enough that you can't eat, you may think, "I shouldn't take insulin today." Nothing could be more wrong. Your body is producing extra glucose even though you aren't feeding it.

How to Prevent DKA

Rule One: If your blood glucose level is above 240 mg/dl several times in a row in the same day, check your urine for ketones. But maybe your blood glucose monitor is malfunctioning, or your test strips have gone bad. So recalibrate your meter or try a new bottle of strips.

Rule Two: Anytime you feel queasy or you're vomiting, check your urine for ketones, even if your blood glucose doesn't test high. A build-up of ketones can cause nausea. Don't assume that you're throwing up only because of a stomach bug. And anytime you're sick enough to be home in bed, even if you're not vomiting, check your urine for ketones and your blood glucose levels about every four hours. Parents, anytime your child complains of a stomachache, check his or her urine for ketones. Pregnant women need to test for ketones every day.

You can buy a ketone testing kit at your pharmacy. You don't need a prescription. Don't wait until you're sick to get one. Keep one in your house and check the expiration date every six months.

A typical ketone test kit gives results as: negative, trace, small, moderate, or large.

Trace or small. If you're sick with the flu and your urine shows trace or small amounts of ketones, that's not so bad. Even people who don't have diabetes show ketones in their urine when they're sick. Follow your sick-day plan, which includes drinking plenty of fluids, and check your blood glucose and ketones again in three to four hours.

Moderate or large. If your urine has moderate or large amounts of ketones, check your blood glucose level and call your doctor immediately. You'll probably need to take extra rapid- or short-acting insulin. Or ask your health care team in advance what you

---

RECOMMENDED

A yearly flu shot is recommended for any person with diabetes who is over 6 months old.

An adult with diabetes should have a pneumococcal vaccination at least once in his or her lifetime.

---

should do (especially regarding insulin). This way you can take action on your own.

If you don't realize that ketones are building up and take steps to reverse it, you can develop DKA. If it's a mild case, you'll need treatment in an outpatient clinic. If it's more serious, you'll be hospitalized.

Symptoms of DKA

Nausea and vomiting
Loss of appetite
Abdominal pain
Thirst
Weakness
Visual disturbances
Sleepiness

Signs That Others Might Notice

Warm, dry skin
Rapid, deep breathing; sighing
Fruity odor on breath

HOME SWEET HOME

At the age of 35, I have moved into my own apartment for the first time. I've had roommates since college, mostly for financial reasons. Housing isn't cheap where I live, even for professionals who make a decent living. (Of course, the plan was to have been married by now, but that's another story.)

I just love my place. I have a big bedroom, an office, a spacious living room and dining room area, and three huge closets with built-in shelves. My neighborhood is fabulous, filled with dozens of restaurants, shops, and clubs just a short walk away. Because my building is 40 years old, the rent is lower than for many of the other apartments in the area.

Best of all, it's mine. I'm having a ball decorating it exactly the way I want, with furniture I've picked up at house sales, photos of friends and family lining the walls, and beloved art deco items scattered throughout. I've got my books, TV and VCR, and computer hooked up to the Internet. It's my own little heavenly piece of the universe!

But a nagging thought keeps bringing me back to earth: I have type 1 diabetes; is it really okay for me to be living alone?

Generally, I don't have any major problems with hypoglycemia. I do have a lot of low sugars, but I almost always feel my symptoms and treat myself. When I drop low at night, I wake up. Except for that one night at a holiday party back in December 1997. In the course of the evening I drank almost four beers. The next morning, my roommate found me lying on the floor of my room, babbling incoherently. She called 911. When the paramedics tested my glucose, it was below 20 mg/dl.

I now know that I cannot drink that much again. While alcohol may raise blood sugar initially, its long-term effect is to lower it. Now that I'm living alone, I might have one or two drinks when I go out, but I'm sure to also eat food, and I'll ask a friend to call me the next day to make sure I'm okay.

My mother, who lives in another city, suggested that I give a spare key to my next-door neighbor, who happens to be a paramedic. That seems like a good idea, but we've only said "hi" a couple times. I can't picture myself knocking on his door one evening and saying, "Hi, I'm your new neighbor. I have diabetes, so would you please check on me every morning, and if I don't answer, come into my apartment and give me orange juice?"

My doctor believes that an insulin pump is the answer. I am considering it, but I have major reservations about wearing something on my body at all times. Also, I'm not convinced that a pump would result in less hypoglycemia than my current regimen.

Meantime I've given my co-workers the phone number of my rental managers, who have keys to my apartment. If I'm not at work by 10:30, my office will call them, and they will check on me and give me juice if I need it. I was very nervous when I initially explained my situation to the husband and wife who manage the building, fearing that they would not react well and consider me a troublesome tenant. I was relieved when

Mr. M. told me that both of his parents—rest their souls—also had diabetes. "My mother used to carry glucose tablets in her purse," he told me.

But that doesn't cover weekends, or on days when I'm not scheduled to be in the office. Those are precisely the times when I'm at greater risk because my schedule is different.

I've concluded that what I'm supposed to do is just what I've been doing: cutting down on my drinking (a good idea for other reasons!), asking friends to call if necessary, and always testing my blood sugar before bed and eating a snack if it's less than 100 mg/dl.

Is that enough? I hope so. I've decided that it's worth the risk. We have to live our lives in the best ways we know how. If I get to a point where I can't feel my hypo symptoms, I may have to rethink things. But for now, as I look around my comfy little haven, I know I've made the right decision.

Miriam E. Tucker
Diabetes Forecast
February 2000

Staying Active

Staying active is the fun part of diabetes management. Any way you do it—walk, jump, jog, ride, skate, bike, climb, ski, or chase the ball—you defend yourself against heart disease. When you're fit, you feel better, you look better, and your body works better.

You don't have to run a marathon to be fit. As many ways as people play, that's how many ways there are to gain fitness. Play daily and you're on your way. All you need is a fitness plan based on your health and needs.

Tell Me Again, Why Exercise?

Most important is this: People who exercise are less likely to have heart attacks. This is particularly important for you because people with diabetes have a higher risk of heart attack.

Regular exercise strengthens your heart and circulatory system. Active movement gets your heart pumping and improves the flow of blood through your small blood vessels. Exercise helps decrease "bad" cholesterol, increase "good" cholesterol, and lowers blood pressure.

As with everyone, exercise improves physical health and mental attitude. It helps you lose body fat. It's important in preserving bone strength and preventing osteoporosis in women. It's a great stress reliever. It's fun!

Before You Start Something New . . .

To help gain benefits from exercise with few drawbacks, it's wise to get the advice of your health care team when you start or change an exercise program. You may need a physical exam. Almost certainly you will need advice from a dietitian on adjusting food and insulin.

Although almost everyone with diabetes can and should exercise, some activities may be better for you than others. If you have eye disease, kidney disease, nerve damage, or blood vessel disease, you may need to avoid certain kinds of exercises.

If you're over 35 or have heart disease, you'll need an electrocardiogram, which looks at heart function, before your doctor gives the go-ahead. Your doctor may ask you to take an exercise stress test to look at how your heart and blood pressure react to a work-out. For this test, your doctor may want to refer you to an exercise physiologist. Exercise physiologists conduct treadmill tests or bicycle testing while checking your blood pressure and heart function. They also figure out your percent of body fat, and test your strength, flexibility, and endurance. Based on this information, they develop exercise programs to fit your schedule and special needs.

Consult with your health care team to find your answers to these questions:

- How often shall I exercise?
- How long shall my exercise session be?
- How hard shall I exercise, and how will I judge this? Should I count my heart rate? How do I do that? What heart rate should I aim for?
- Are there any types of exercise I should avoid?
- Are there any symptoms (for hypo-glycemia or heart disease) I should watch out for?
- Are there special precautions I should take?
- Do I take less insulin or change my injection site before I exercise?

Your Main Concern: Changes in Blood Glucose

Your muscles use glucose for energy. When you first start exercising, your body uses stored glucose in the muscles and liver for fuel. As this runs low, your body looks to blood glucose for fuel. So, during exercise, blood glucose levels can fall. Then after you

stop exercising, your body restores glucose
to the muscles and liver by taking glucose
from the blood, which further lowers blood
glucose levels. This goes on for hours after
exercise.

Don't forget that the body can absorb
insulin differently from day to day. This
means that the same amount of insulin can
have effects that differ from one day to the
next. And exercise is known to increase
blood flow, which can also increase how fast
the insulin you inject starts to work.

Because exercise lowers blood glucose
levels and can speed insulin in its work lowering blood glucose levels, it's a good idea to
test your blood glucose level when you exercise. Otherwise, you may have a low blood
glucose reaction without expecting it.

Here are some guidelines that will help
keep blood glucose in line with exercise:

- **Low.** If your blood glucose level is less
  than 100 mg/dl before exercise, have a
  snack that contains 15 grams of carbohydrate and test again 15–30 minutes later.
  For example, fruit, juice, half a sandwich,
  crackers, or cereal would fit the bill.
- **In range.** If your blood glucose level is
  100–250 mg/dl, exercise. Until you learn
  the effects of exercise on your body,
  self-monitor your blood glucose during
  and after exercise to see whether you
  need a snack.
- **High.** If your blood glucose is over
  250 mg/dl, test your urine for ketones. If
  ketones are high, this means you don't
  have enough insulin. You'll need another

injection. Don't exercise until ketone levels return to negative or trace amounts. If your blood glucose is over 300 mg/dl, even without ketones, be cautious with exercise. It may raise glucose higher.

■ **Check first.** It's good to know which way your blood glucose level is heading, especially if you're about to start an activity where you can't easily "pull over," such as scuba diving, sailing, or skiing. Check your blood glucose 1 hour before and then again 30 minutes before you start. If your blood glucose level is heading down, even if the latest test says it's in the safe range, you may want a snack to keep it from going any lower.

■ **Know when your insulins are active.** Try not to exercise when your insulin is peaking unless you've eaten.

■ **How fast?** Realize that if you inject insulin into a muscle that you then use for exercise, the insulin may be absorbed more quickly.

■ **Snack.** Eat an extra amount of carbohydrate (10–15 grams) after 30 minutes of exercise if you plan to continue exercising and if the exercise requires endurance, such as running, aerobics, squash, or racquetball. Have a snack for every additional hour that you exercise.

If the exercise is very intense and long, such as a marathon, you may need to eat 15 grams of carbohydrate every 15–30 minutes. Good snack choices are foods high in carbohydrate and low in fat, such as fig bars or yogurt rather than candy bars. Fresh fruit, which has a high water content, is also a good choice.

▓ **If you feel a low blood glucose reaction** coming on while exercising, stop exercising. Don't make the mistake of thinking you can last a little while longer. Check your blood glucose. If it's low, take some form of sugar. Some fruit juice or a regular (nondiet) soft drink will provide sugar as well as replace water lost during exercise.

▓ **Always carry** some glucose gels or tablets, raisins, or hard candy just in case you need it when exercising.

▓ **Keep hydrated.** Dehydration affects blood glucose levels. Drink before you're thirsty. Drink water for the first hour or so. Then have watery drinks, such as diluted juice.

▓ **Wear medical identification.**

▓ **Exercise with someone.** If you're going to exercise alone, at least let someone know where you are and when you expect to be back, and carry a cell phone or change for a phone call.

▓ **Remember, exercise lowers blood glucose for up to 24 hours** after you stop working out. Monitor your blood glucose levels to prevent yourself from having a low blood glucose reaction.

Adapting to Your Own Needs

Some people reduce their insulin dose before exercising instead of eating extra food. If you exercise hard for about an hour, you may want to reduce the insulin that is active at that time by about 20%.

If you exercise longer than an hour (long-distance cycling, hiking), you may want to reduce both your short- or rapid-acting insulin and your longer-acting insulin.

If your blood glucose level is highest in the morning, try exercising after breakfast. If you like to exercise before dinner, see whether you need an afternoon snack before you exercise. If you are an evening exerciser, you may decide to reduce your insulin before dinner, have a larger dinner, or plan a snack during exercise or at bedtime.

Listen to your body. You should not have too much fatigue, pain, or shortness of breath during your work-out. Doing too much too fast can lead to injuries that may keep you from doing anything at all.

People with diabetes are at risk for foot problems. Wear good athletic shoes and socks that wick away moisture. Check your feet after you exercise for red spots or blisters.

If you're inactive now, start with a little activity every day. With time, you can work up to a good aerobic program. A work-out session has 5–10 minutes of warm-up exercises and stretching, followed by 20–30 minutes of aerobic exercise, and finally 5–10 minutes of cool-down exercises and stretching. Daily stretching will increase your flexibility. To see improvement in your fitness level, work out at least five times a week.

LEAVING DIABETES IN THE DUST

Is there ever a time when anyone with type 1 diabetes can, more or less, forget about it? Even just for a little while?

I've discovered you can.

Last February, my friend and fellow French classmate, Kate, asked me if I was going to participate with Webster on Wheels. My first question was, "What is Webster on Wheels?"

"It's this bicycling trip that Brian [our French professor] is leading this summer," she replied. "I think it will be great. We ride our bikes all through the south of France and through the Pyrenees Mountains. We'll get to go through different towns and meet people. What better way to see a country than to bike through it and really experience it?"

I pondered the idea. The more I thought about it, the more excited I got. However, I was faced with two problems: how to fund the trip and how to manage my diabetes on a 19-day minimalist biking trip.

The money part was easy. I was scheduled to get my bachelor's degree in May, so I requested this trip as my graduation gift. My parents and grandparents agreed.

The diabetes issue, though, was another story— 19 days, camping every night, no accompanying vehicle, 1,800 cubic inches of storage. How was I going to pull this off? My fears would not stop me, however. This was something I wanted to do, needed to do, and was going to do.

In late March, I went on an insulin pump. I knew that being on a pump would be advantageous on a trip such as this. The pump manufacturer gave me some helpful hints and information, which helped with making dosage adjustments for exercise. Once I became stabilized on the pump, I began some light training on my bike.

Two weeks before my departure, I told my endocrinologist and her nurse about my trip. They were ten times more worried than I was. They were worried about the possibility of my pump breaking and/or my insulin going bad from heat while my only concern was low blood sugar from heavy activity.

I made sure that I went prepared. My diabetic supplies consisted of three bottles of Humalog for my pump, one bottle of NPH in case of pump breakage, a meter, tons of extra pump supplies, plenty of test strips, and about ten pounds of various brands of energy bars. To allay my initial concerns about low blood sugars, I decided to lower my basal rate while I was riding. Also, I would cut the boluses by half and just eat extra meals. As you can tell, I thought my diabetes was going to be a huge problem during the trip.

I could not have been more wrong.

On July 28, three other students, our professor, and I arrived in Bordeaux, France. We reassembled our bikes and started on our way. Within an hour, rain began pouring down. That didn't matter. We had no choice but to get to the campsite in Arcachon before dark.

We averaged 24 to 36 miles a day, and on one particular day we covered about 80 miles. There were a few rest days, but for the most part we rode our bikes a lot! We biked in rain, blazing sun, and strong winds. We rode on flat land, up hills, down hills, and through mountains. We even biked to the airport at 4 a.m. by the light of two flashlights.

In spite of all that, we had an amazing time. We met a lot of kind and interesting people, many of whom were merchants and campground owners. We sampled delicious pastries, baguettes, and cheeses. We saw historic castles and cemeteries. But most important of all, we pushed ourselves to do something well beyond our comfort zones.

This trip pushed me mentally, physically, and spiritually. It also scared me to death at times.

After completing the trip, I read over my journal to see just how much, in retrospect, my diabetes had encumbered me. The only thing I found that remotely related to my diabetes was a running record of my blood sugar readings. The exercise did wonders for my blood sugar and, surprisingly, I was low only a few times.

I was surprised to find that the bulk of my journal passages contained accounts of what I saw, did, and how I felt. It wasn't about me and my diabetes. It was about me as a person, active and full of purpose. It was me having a fantastic and unforgettable experience.

Of course, the diabetes never went away, nor did I ignore it. But it never dominated my experience, never got in the way. I found I could be free to challenge myself, to explore, to experience new worlds.

While it was impossible for me to forget my diabetes completely, I realized that despite it, I could still do anything I wish to do. Even though there were many obstacles to overcome, I was able to have the experience of a lifetime.

Amy Knese
Diabetes Forecast
March 2000

Diabetes Complications

Diabetes is complicated enough—without the thought of complications in the future. Complications are health problems related to diabetes. The ones most people think of as being diabetes complications are kidney disease (nephropathy), diabetic eye disease (retinopathy), nerve damage (neuropathy), and foot ulcers leading to amputation. Less well known is that people with diabetes are at higher risk for heart attack and stroke.

Maybe you shrug your shoulders and say there's no point in looking ahead to health problems. After all, complications don't strike everyone with type 1 diabetes, and it's not easy to think about such troubles.

But there's good reason to think ahead. If you make changes in your life now, you'll lower your chances of getting complications by more than 50% down the road.

You can start with the ABCs.

A1C

A1C is a measure of your overall blood glucose control. (See pp. 56–59.) The closer your A1C is to the normal (nondiabetic) level, the lower your risk of diabetic eye, kidney, and nerve disease. Any improvement in your A1C level lowers your risk. If your A1C is 10% now and you get it down to 9%, you've lowered your risk. If you get it below 7% without too many episodes of hypoglycemia per week, you're doing well.

Blood Pressure

High blood pressure increases your risk of heart disease, stroke, and diabetic eye disease. Poorly controlled blood pressure is a major factor in the progression of diabetic kidney disease.

As dangerous as high blood pressure can be, you'll probably have no symptoms. That's why it's called the silent killer.

You want to keep your blood pressure below 130/80.

Cholesterol

People talk about their "cholesterol levels." Doctors call these fats in the blood "lipids." HDL cholesterol is **H**ealthy; you want the number **H**igh. LDL cholesterol is bad; you want the number **L**ow. Triglycerides, another type of blood fat, are also bad. You want the level low, too.

Type of lipid	Goal
HDL ("good") cholesterol	For men: over 45 mg/dl
	For women: over 55 mg/dl
LDL ("bad") cholesterol	Under 100 mg/dl
Triglycerides	Under 150 mg/dl

Those are the goals—now how can you achieve them?

Don't smoke. You probably already know that smoking can cause a wide and frightening range of lung disorders. Smoking also raises blood pressure. It damages your heart and circulatory system by narrowing your blood vessels over time. The damage contributes to heart disease, impotence, amputation, and kidney disease.

Have you tried to quit? Don't give up! Most smokers quit four times before staying quit. Have you already tried a quit-smoking class, going cold turkey, using nicotine gum or patches? Consider hypnosis or acupuncture. Ask your doctor about bupropion (Zyban). Zyban is a prescription medication that doesn't contain nicotine but can help you quit smoking. You can use it along with nicotine patches or gum.

Eat healthy foods. A healthy meal plan has little saturated fat and cholesterol; lots of whole grains, fruits, and vegetables; and a moderate amount of protein. Eating wisely reduces your risk of cardiovascular disease and some cancers.

Stay active. Regular physical activity helps keep your blood pressure down, improves your cholesterol levels, helps you achieve and maintain a healthy weight, strengthens your heart, and reduces stress. Do some physical activity every day. Find ways to make it a daily habit. Get off the elevator one floor early. Park further away. Start a garden. Take a swimming class. Walk around the block after lunch.

Take it easy on the salt. Excess sodium may contribute to high blood pressure. Keep your sodium intake below 2,400 mg per day. If you have kidney disease, ask your doctor what your sodium limit is.

Watch your alcohol intake. Alcohol can make other medical problems worse. Avoid alcohol if you have:

■ *High blood pressure.* Alcohol makes your blood pressure increase. If you already have high blood pressure, cutting out even light alcohol consumption may reduce your blood pressure.

▓ *Neuropathy*. Alcohol is directly toxic to nerves. If you have peripheral nerve damage in your arms or legs, heavy or regular drinking can increase pain, numbness, and other symptoms. There is some evidence that even regular light drinking (less than two drinks per week) is harmful.

▓ *Gastric problems*. Alcohol can increase the discomfort of chronic bowel problems such as diabetic diarrhea or constipation.

▓ *Retinopathy*. Heavy drinking (three or more drinks a day) is associated with the development and progression of eye disease.

▓ *High triglycerides*. Alcohol affects the clearance of fat from the blood by the liver and encourages the liver to produce more triglycerides. Even moderate amounts of alcohol (two 4-oz glasses of wine a week) can raise your triglyceride levels.

▓ *Other complications*. These include liver disease, pancreatitis, some heart or kidney diseases. And, of course, don't drink if you're pregnant.

Relax. Doing something you enjoy just 20 minutes twice a day can relieve everyday stress and tension that can contribute to high blood pressure.

Take your medications. High blood pressure and high cholesterol don't make you feel bad, so taking medication doesn't make you feel better. You may even have side effects from taking the medications. All in all, it's sometimes hard to keep taking some of the medicines that have been prescribed for you.

■ *Remind yourself* that even though high blood pressure and high cholesterol don't make you feel bad, they are leading you closer to heart attack, stroke, and other complications.

■ *Keep track* of your lab results so you can see that the medications are actually doing you good.

■ *If side effects* make you want to stop taking your medication, report this to your pharmacist or doctor. You may be able to take another medication that will do the job with fewer side effects.

■ *If the cost* of the medication is making you skip pills, tell your pharmacist or doctor. There may be a generic version available, or a less expensive medication that will work for you.

Treatments for Complications

All your hard work can't guarantee you will be free of complications. Factors you don't control—such as your age, your race, and your genes—influence your risk.

If you get a complication, you may have many of the same feelings you had when you were first diagnosed with type 1 diabetes— anger, fear, guilt, or denial. You may have thought that you had good diabetes control all figured out, and it's frustrating to find you now have to make another effort. You may feel overwhelmed that on top of the ordinary stresses of life and having diabetes, you have new health problems to contend with.

Treatments for diabetes complications are more effective every year. Don't listen too closely to information about complications from friends or relatives. They may remember therapies from years ago, and they don't know about modern ones.

The rest of this chapter explains some of the most common complications of diabetes, and ways to prevent them and treat them.

Cardiovascular Disease

Cardiovascular disease can go by many names—arteriosclerosis, hardening of the arteries, peripheral vascular disease, coronary artery disease, and stroke—but they all describe problems with the heart and circulatory system. The flow of blood through the body provides all the oxygen, glucose, and other substances needed to run your body and keep its cells alive.

Narrowing or clogging of blood vessels, called arteriosclerosis, limits blood flow and can kill tissues. People with diabetes are more likely to get arteriosclerosis.

Diabetes also seems to change blood chemistry, making heart disease more likely. Diabetes changes the number and make-up of proteins that deliver lipids to cells. These lipoproteins will usually return to normal if you achieve good control. Diabetes also affects blood cells known as platelets. They may produce too much of a chemical that constricts blood vessels and causes clotting. And, to add insult to injury, once an artery is

An Aspirin a Day?

An aspirin a day lowers the risk of heart attack and stroke.

Who should take aspirin?

■ Men and women with a history of heart attack, bypass surgery, stroke or TIAs (transient ischemic attacks), peripheral vascular disease, claudication (pain in legs when walking), or angina.

■ Men and women with one or more risk factors for cardiovascular disease:

- Family history of coronary heart disease
- Cigarette smoking
- High blood pressure
- Obesity
- Protein in the urine (microalbuminuria or proteinuria)
- Total cholesterol over 200 mg/dl
- LDL cholesterol 100 mg/dl or more
- HDL cholesterol less than 45 mg/dl (men), or less than 55 mg/dl (women)
- Triglycerides more than 200 mg/dl

■ Age over 30

What dose?
Use enteric-coated aspirin in doses of
81-325 mg/day. Ask your doctor.

Who shouldn't?
Aspirin therapy isn't right for you if
you have aspirin allergy, bleeding ten-
dency, anticoagulant therapy, recent
gastrointestinal bleeding, clinically
active liver disease, or if you are under
the age of 21 (because of the risk of
Reye's syndrome).

damaged, poor blood flow due to uncon-
trolled diabetes can slow its healing.

Cardiovascular disease can cut off
blood supply to the heart and brain. If blood
to the heart is slowed for a time, the pain that
results is called angina. A complete, long-
lasting stoppage of blood is a heart attack.
When blood to the brain is stopped, a stroke
results. When blood in the arteries in the legs
is blocked, the leg pain that goes along with
walking is called intermittent claudication.

Treatment

If you develop cardiovascular disease, the
four ways to prevent a heart attack—stop
smoking, eat a healthy diet, control blood
pressure, and exercise—can still help you.
They may slow or stop the progression of
the disease. A diet low in cholesterol and
saturated fat is especially good. Eating more
fiber lowers your levels of "bad"
cholesterol.

When these measures fail, surgery is possible to open blocked blood vessels. Balloon angioplasty uses a balloon at the tip of a tube to open the vessels. The surgeon inflates the balloon where the artery is blocked to open up the vessel. Arthrectomy opens the blockage by boring a hole through it. Laser surgery melts away blockages with an intense beam of light. These surgeries require little recovery time.

A more severe blockage calls for more serious surgery. Arterial bypass surgery creates a detour for blood to flow around the blockage. Surgeons remove part of a large artery from the chest wall or a vein from the leg and sew it above and below the blocked segment. Blood flows through the new vessel instead of the blocked one.

There are treatments for most other types of cardiovascular disease too. Intermittent claudication may be relieved by exercise, drug therapy, or surgery. Strokes usually call for a combination approach: normalizing blood glucose, blood pressure, and blood lipid levels; helping the person recover mental and physical abilities; and giving drugs to control blood clotting. Sometimes, surgery is needed. Treatment of angina aims at reducing the amount of oxygen the heart tissue requires and increasing the oxygen going to the heart. People with diabetes and angina are advised to get more exercise, normalize their blood glucose levels, and lose weight. They also may take medication or need surgery.

Retinopathy

Retinopathy is a disease of the tiny blood vessels that supply the retinas, the "movie screens" at the back of your eyes where the images you see are projected. When it begins, you don't notice diabetic retinopathy. It takes an exam by an eye doctor to see the changes in the blood vessels. Detected early, retinopathy can be slowed or stopped altogether.

In one form of diabetic retinopathy, blood vessels may close off or weaken and leak blood, fluid, and fat into the eye. This form is called *nonproliferative (background) retinopathy*. It may lead to blurry vision, but it usually does not cause blindness.

"Thank God I had been going for eye check-ups routinely, because they caught it at an early stage."
–Bill Davidson

Nonproliferative retinopathy can progress to a more serious, rarer condition called *proliferative retinopathy*. When this happens, new blood vessels sprout in the retina. That may sound good, but the new vessels grow out of control. They are fragile, so they rupture easily with high blood pressure, exercise, vomiting from morning sickness, or even while sleeping. Blood may leak into the fluid-filled portion of the eye in front of the retina, impairing sight. Scar tissue may form on the retina as well. When the scar tissue shrinks, it can pull the retinal layers apart. This damages sight; images look as though they are projected on a sheet flapping in the breeze. Glaucoma may go along with proliferative retinopathy. This increased pressure in the eye can be treated if it is spotted early on.

Retinopathy can also affect the macula of the eye, the central portion of the retina that gives us sharp vision for seeing fine detail. The swelling of the macula, called macular edema, can limit vision and lead to blindness.

After 20 years of diabetes, nearly all people with type 1 diabetes have some degree of retinopathy.

Catch It Early

Long before vision is affected by diabetes, tiny changes occur in the retina. If these changes are caught early, they can be treated so that your vision isn't affected.

Your primary care physician will look into your eyes during your yearly physical exams, but you also need a more thorough exam by an eye doctor—an ophthalmologist or an optometrist. You need a **dilated eye exam**. It goes like this:

The eye doctor puts drops in your eyes to dilate (open up) your pupils. You're sent back to the waiting room. You'll start to have trouble focusing. For example, you may not be able to read the magazine that you had been reading just before you got the drops.

After about a half an hour, you're brought back into the exam room and the doctor uses a strong light to look into your eyes and examine your retinas.

When you're leaving the office, because your pupils are dilated, you'll be told to wear sunglasses on the way home. If you don't have any, you may be given disposable sunglasses.

If the above description doesn't sound familiar to you, you have not had a dilated eye exam. Make an appointment with an eye doctor today. Don't wait for your primary care doctor to suggest it. Studies show that many doctors fail to remind their patients with diabetes to have eye exams. And don't wait until you have trouble with your eyes. You can have severe, sight-threatening changes in your retinas without having any symptoms.

If you are:	Have a dilated eye exam:	Have follow-up exams:
Under 10 years old	Ask your doctor if you need one	
10 to 29 years old	Within 3 to 5 years of diagnosis	Once a year
30 years or older	When you are diagnosed with diabetes	Once a year
Trying to get pregnant	Now (before you conceive)	As directed by doctor
Pregnant	Now (in first trimester)	As directed by doctor

Treatment

The best treatment for people with diabetes in danger of losing their sight involves a laser—an intense beam of light. An ophthalmologist aims the laser at the retina to create hundreds of tiny burns that destroy abnormal blood vessels, patch leaky ones, and slow the formation of new fragile vessels. This procedure is called photocoagulation. In people with high-risk proliferative retinopathy or macular edema, photocoagulation can usually prevent blindness.

Photocoagulation may not work if the retina has bled a lot or has detached. In these cases, surgery called vitrectomy can remove the blood and scar tissue, stop bleeding, replace some of the vitreous (the clear, jelly-like fluid in the eye) with salt solution, and repair the detached retina.

If you need either of these procedures, choose an ophthalmologist who specializes in retinal disease and has patients with diabetes. And remember that the earlier the procedure is done, the better.

If laser treatment or vitrectomy fail to restore vision, low-vision aids can often help people regain the ability to read the paper, do paperwork, or watch TV.

If you have retinopathy, discuss your exercise program with your eye doctor. Some activities can raise the pressure inside your eyes and lead to bleeding in the retina. Also, avoid taking birth control pills because they may affect the clotting of your blood or increase your blood pressure.

Nephropathy

Your kidneys work 24 hours a day to cleanse your blood of toxic substances made

New Pancreas?

A successful pancreas transplantation will cure your diabetes. However, it is major surgery, which carries some risk. In addition, a pancreas transplant requires lifelong treatment with drugs that suppress the immune system to prevent rejection of the new pancreas. Such drugs are quite strong and have side effects.

The American Diabetes Association recommends the following:

1. Pancreas transplantation should be considered in patients with imminent or established end-stage renal disease (kidney failure) who have had or plan to have a kidney transplant. The person will be on immunosuppression therapy for the kidney transplant. Therefore, a new pancreas adds a lot of benefit for little additional risk.

2. If a kidney transplantation is not needed, pancreas transplantation should be considered only in patients who have: 1) a history of frequent and severe hypoglycemia, hyperglycemia, or ketoacidosis requiring medical attention; 2) clinical and emotional problems with insulin therapy that are so severe as to be incapacitating; and 3) consistent failure of insulin-based management to prevent acute complications.

3. Pancreatic islet cell transplants hold significant potential advantages over whole-gland transplants. However, at this time, islet cell transplantation is an experimental procedure, also requiring immunosuppression, and should be performed only within the setting of controlled research studies.

by or taken into the body. These toxins enter the kidney by crossing the walls of small blood vessels that border it. In people with nephropathy, these blood vessels, called capillaries, cease to be good filters. They become blocked and leakier at the same time. As a result, some wastes that should be removed stay in the blood, and some protein that should stay in the blood is removed and lost in the urine.

Some people with newly diagnosed type 1 diabetes may have an excess of protein in their urine temporarily. But more obvious symptoms of kidney disease take a long time to appear. The kidneys have so much extra filtering ability that 80% of the kidney must be damaged before noticeable problems appear.

Progression

In the early stages of kidney disease, very small amounts of protein leak into the urine. This condition is called microalbuminuria (micro = small, albumin = protein, uria = urine). In those who develop it, microalbuminuria occurs after 5 to 15 years of diabetes. It is one of the earliest stages of kidney disease that can be detected.

Several years after a person has microalbuminuria (mi-cro-al-byu-min-UR-i-a), the kidneys begin to spill larger amounts of protein. At this point, the person is said to have clinical proteinuria and overt nephropathy.

As damage to the filters increases, poisons that are normally removed by the kidneys build up in the blood.

Catch It Early

If you know you have microalbuminuria, you and your doctor can take steps to slow the progression. *If* you know.

You should be tested for microalbuminuria every year once you have had diabetes for five years.

Your doctor may have already tested you for proteinuria. This can be done with a standard urine dipstick test in your doctor's office. If the test is positive, you should have the more sensitive test that can detect microalbuminuria.

Your doctor can screen for microalbuminuria by testing a sample of your urine in the office. The ratio of albumin to creatinine (a waste product) is determined. Normal is less than 30 mg albumin per 1 gram creatinine.

Your doctor might ask you to collect your urine for a certain amount of time: for 4 hours, or overnight, or for 24 hours. It is then tested. Normal is less than 30 mg albumin in 24 hours; microalbuminuria is 30–300 mg; proteinuria is more than 300 mg.

Other stresses to your body, such as an infection or fever, may cause the test to be positive. Therefore, if one test is positive, you will be retested. If two out of three tests in 3–6 months are positive, then you know you have microalbuminuria, and treatment should be started.

If you haven't been tested for microalbuminuria, the next time you see your doctor, arrange to have it done. Don't wait for your doctor to bring it up. In a survey of 1,000 primary care doctors, almost half did not test their patients with diabetes for microalbuminuria.

Treatment

If you are found to have microalbuminuria, you and your doctor will redouble efforts to get your blood pressure down. Even if you don't have high blood pressure, you may be prescribed an ACE inhibitor. ACE inhibitors are blood pressure medications that also preserve kidney function.

You may be advised to lower the amount of protein in your diet.

Very advanced kidney disease means that filtration is greatly disrupted and the kidneys are failing. This condition is end stage renal disease. At this point, there are only two treatment options: dialysis and kidney transplantation.

Neuropathy

Too much blood glucose damages the nervous system. Damaged nerves either can't send messages, send them at the wrong time, or send them too slowly. (The brain and spinal cord are not affected.)

Researchers still aren't sure why high blood glucose harms nerves. It's possible that glucose-coated proteins damage nerves, or high levels of glucose may upset the chemical balance inside nerves. The damage can be indirect, if the blood supply to the nerves is limited and nerves don't receive enough oxygen.

Types and Treatments

Peripheral neuropathy with pain. Neuropathy can strike nerves in the hands and feet. You may feel shooting or stabbing pains, burning, tingling or prickling, or weakness.

Treatment. The pain of peripheral neuropathy will often vanish after a few months or a year of good blood glucose control. Your doctor can prescribe various medications that may relieve pain. These include antidepressants and antiepileptic drugs. A cream made from an extract of hot peppers may work for people who don't respond to other treatments. Sometimes the pain will get worse as your blood sugar levels improve. Keep on because the pain will go away eventually, and your health will be much improved.

Less than two-thirds of people with known diabetes have an annual dilated eye exam.

Men develop diabetes-related vision problems more rapidly than women.

One-fourth to one-half of deaths in people 30 or older with type 1 diabetes of long duration are caused by cardio-vascular disease.

By one account, 54% of people with type 1 diabetes have peripheral neuropathy.

Nearly 13% of men with type 1 diabetes have erectile dysfunction.

A 1993 study of people with diabetic kidney disease found that treatment with an ACE inhibitor cut the risk of death, dialysis, or transplant in half.

People with diabetic retinopathy or macular degeneration can reduce their chances of becoming blind by nearly 90% if they receive early laser surgery.

Peripheral neuropathy with numbness.
Sensory nerves tell you when you're touching a hot pot, when your hands are cold, when your shoe is rubbing your skin raw. Neuropathy can affect these nerves resulting in "loss of protective sensation." You aren't able to sense heat and cold, which increases your risk of burns and frostbite.

Loss of protective sensation puts you at risk for amputation. You may not feel the pain of a blister or small cut on your foot. The small cut on your foot goes untreated. It may get infected and progress to an ulcer. If a lower-limb infection goes out of control, a surgeon may need to remove part of the foot or leg to save the rest of the leg from becoming infected.

Amputation is frightening, but it does not mean the end of a normal lifestyle. It's not even the end of walking. The surgeon will remove as little of the limb as possible so that walking will be less difficult. After the limb heals, a prosthesis will be fitted. New prosthetic limbs are lighter and more comfortable than the clunky models of the past.

Catch It Early

If you know you have lost protective sensation, you'll know to be extra careful about your feet. You'll check your feet every day for irritations. You'll wear good athletic shoes rather than tight, pointy-toed shoes that may give you blisters. You'll have a health care professional examine your feet every three months.

Your doctor can test you for loss of protective sensation by using what's called a monofilament. It looks like a long bristle from a paint brush. Your doctor touches it to various places on the bottom of your foot. If you can't feel the touch, you have lost protective sensation.

Monofilament testing should be part of a yearly exam of your feet. If your doctor or nurse hasn't tested you and doesn't seem to know what you're talking about, you can get your own monofilament for free and have a family member test you. Call Health Resources and Services Administration at 1-888-ASK-HRSA (1-888-275-4772). Via the internet, go to the Lower Extremity Amputation Prevention Program web site at http://bphc.hrsa.gov/leap.

Focal neuropathy. A rarer condition, focal neuropathy, centers on a single nerve or group of nerves. It may arise when blood supply to a nerve shuts off because a vessel becomes blocked. It may also happen when a nerve becomes squeezed. It can injure nerves that sense touch and pain as well as nerves responsible for moving muscles. Fortunately, it usually goes away fairly fast, within 2 weeks to 18 months after better blood glucose control is achieved.

Carpal tunnel syndrome is one focal neuropathy seen more often in people with diabetes. The median nerve of the forearm can be squeezed in its passageway, or tunnel, by the carpal bones at the wrist. The syndrome is three times more common in women than in men. It may cause tingling, burning, and numbness so that you may drop objects. Fortunately, carpal tunnel syndrome is not permanent. You can treat it with good blood glucose control, medications, or surgery to remove tissues squeezing the nerve.

Autonomic neuropathy. Neuropathy can damage nerves that you don't control voluntarily, such as those to your internal organs. This condition is called autonomic neuropathy. It may slow down stomach and gut muscles, leading to constipation, a feeling of fullness, diarrhea, nausea, or occasional vomiting.

Damaged nerves to the bladder may cause muscle weakness so that it can't get completely empty. Then the bladder will occasionally empty involuntarily. Because urine remains in the bladder for a long time, it can cause urinary tract infections.

Men may slowly lose the ability to have an erection, even though they still have sexual desire (see Erectile Dysfunction, p. 45). Women, too, may have decreased sexual response.

Nerves that control blood pressure may be affected; when you stand up, you may feel dizzy or lightheaded. Nerves to the skin may cause too much or too little sweating or very dry skin.

Nerves to the heart may fail to speed up or slow down your heart rate in response to exercise. This is one reason to get a check-up before you begin any program of exercise. If you can't trust your heart rate to reflect your exertion, you will not be able to use standard ways to find a target heart rate during and after a work-out.

Treatment

There are different treatments for the different effects of autonomic neuropathy. Digestive problems take patience and some trial and error to treat. You may be able to avoid them by changing your eating habits. Eat small, frequent meals instead of large ones, and choose lower-fiber and lower-fat foods. Some medications can increase emptying of gut and eliminate the feeling of fullness.

Incontinence, or urine leakage, can be treated with training in bladder control and timed urination by a planned bladder-emptying program. Urinate by the clock every 2 hours rather than waiting for the feeling of fullness. Men may need to urinate sitting down. Applying pressure over the bladder may be helpful. If these steps don't work, taking oral medications, learning to use a catheter, and having surgery can work. Fecal incontinence (passing stool involuntarily) is treated with medicine for diarrhea and biofeedback training.

Sudden drops in blood pressure on standing can be treated as well. You may need to stop drinking alcohol and stop taking certain medications, such as diuretics. Your health care team may advise you to take medications for low blood pressure, raise the salt content of your diet, change your sleeping position, and improve your general health. Be careful when you stand up, and try not to stand still for long periods of time to prevent fainting. When you get up in the morning, sit on the edge of the bed and dangle your feet for 5 minutes before you stand up.

Erectile Dysfunction

Erectile dysfunction (impotence) occurs in more than half of men over age 50 who have diabetes. It can affect younger men as well.

Diabetes can damage nerves and blood vessels. When the nerves are damaged, small blood vessels don't relax, which prevents them from expanding with the flow of blood that makes the penis erect. Rarely, erectile dysfunction occurs when blood vessels are blocked or made narrow because of vascular disease.

Some drugs used to treat high blood pressure, anxiety, depression, peptic ulcers, and painful neuropathy may cause erectile dysfunction in some men. If you take any of these types of drugs and experience erectile dysfunction, tell your doctor. You may be able to switch to a different medication.

Erectile dysfunction is a treatable problem. Because there are many causes and many different treatments, every case has to be assessed individually. If you're experiencing erectile dysfunction, you'll want to have a comprehensive evaluation before any treatment is started.

Treatment

Oral medication. Sildenafil (Viagra) is a pill that can help with erectile dysfunction. About 60 to 70 percent of men with erectile dysfunction respond to sildenafil.

Penile constriction ring. This works for men who can get erections but have problems maintaining them. After you get an erection, you put the constriction ring at the base of your penis and take it off after you've had intercourse.

Vacuum erection. You put the plastic tube over your penis. With a hand- or battery-operated pump, you create a vacuum within the tube. This draws blood into your penis, resulting in an erection. You then put a con-striction ring at the base of your penis to trap the blood.

These devices are quite safe and rela-tively successful. However, they do require a moderate amount of manual dexterity, and some couples find them to be intrusive.

The MUSE System. Using a small plunger device, you insert a small pellet of medica-tion directly into your urethra. The medication—prostaglandin—causes the arteries of the penis to relax. More blood flows into the penis, causing an erection.

Penile self-injection. Using a fine needle, you inject a small amount of medication directly into your penis. The medication causes the blood vessels to expand, bringing extra blood into the penis and causing an erection.

Penile prostheses. One type is a semi-rigid, bendable rod that is surgically implanted into the penis. Another type is a more complex mechanical system of inflatable cylinders.

When an erection is needed, the cylinders are inflated with a pump placed within the scrotum. These prostheses are not popular now. There is a risk of infection and equipment breakdown. When prosthesis malfunction occurs, it usually requires surgical correction.

ME–AN ATHLETE?

It's my turn next.

I glance desperately at the clock as I wipe my sweaty palms against the sides of my scratchy nylon shorts. Too quickly, the volleyball is passed heavily into my hands. My arms feel like limp pasta. I hit the ball with all my might, and it makes a short arc in the air, falling miserably short of the net.

It is this vision of junior high gym class that flashed through my mind as my diabetes educator espoused the benefits of exercise. I could recall the sensation of my stomach plummeting when I would step into the gym and see the volleyball nets set up. I cannot remember one time when my ball made it over the net.

Physical activity was never something I excelled at or even showed interest in. I was more comfortable with my nose in a book than I was running on a track or kicking a soccer ball. Finding out I had type 1 diabetes my sophomore year of college was shocking. But to hear that I needed to begin an exercise program, a lifelong exercise program, was overwhelming. The finger pricks, injections, and diet plan were difficult, but, for me, the true struggle was exercise.

Over the next several years I walked, took aerobics and yoga classes, did fitness tapes, and joined a health club. I would throw myself into a program, stick with it for a couple of weeks, and then get tired of it. My blood sugars would be great while I exercised, but I hated every minute of it. I knew that I needed to make exercise a permanent part of my daily life, but it was a fact I continuously fought.

Until recently.

Last fall a severe case of the flu brought me close to diabetic ketoacidosis, and, as a result, I cut back my work hours so I could make health my priority. I forced myself to do some kind of aerobic activity three times a week, and I started lifting hand weights. During each workout I tried to focus on the positive effects of exercise.

Within a couple of months, I didn't have to convince myself of these effects—I was feeling them. My blood sugars stabilized, my energy and mood soared, and I was developing muscle for the first time in my life. I was stunned. Was this the same person who had quaked in her shoes at the sight of the volleyball nets?

I had convinced myself that since I had never been athletic, I simply wasn't capable of exercise. I had also talked myself into believing that exercise was a horrible ritual to avoid if at all possible. But here I was, growing stronger and more flexible with each workout, and enjoying the pride and feeling of accomplishment that exercise brings. For the first time, I felt in control of my diabetes. My most recent A1C was the lowest it has ever been: 6.7.

At age 26, I am healthier now with diabetes than I ever was without it. I wish I could go back to the volleyball court in junior high gym class. When it came my turn to serve, I would hit the ball with all my might. I have no doubt that it would soar.

Amanda Magoto Prenger
Diabetes Forecast
January 2002

12

Women

From puberty through menopause, your "female" hormones will affect your blood glucose levels.

Menstruation

Some women with diabetes notice that their blood glucose levels are higher in the week before their periods. The reason? The female hormones estrogen and progesterone.

We count the days of a menstrual cycle starting with the first day of bleeding as day 1. Around day 13, estrogen levels go up. Ovulation occurs. Then progesterone levels start to go up. Toward the end of the month, if there is no pregnancy, the levels of estrogen and progesterone start to drop and bleeding starts.

Some studies show that when estrogen and progesterone levels are high, your insulin doesn't work as well. Blood glucose levels creep up. The hormones also cause your liver to release more glucose into your bloodstream. And many women eat more, and more starchy foods, just before their periods. That affects blood glucose, too.

Are your hormones affecting your blood glucose levels? Look at three months worth of your blood glucose logs. Mark the first day of your period for each month, and look at your blood glucose levels the week before. Were they on average higher (or for some women, lower) than in the other three weeks of the month?

You may need a little more insulin to stay within your blood glucose goals the week before your period. Exercise can also help, because it helps insulin work. If you're one of the few women who run low before their periods, you can take less insulin during that week. Talk to your diabetes educator or doctor for guidance on insulin changes.

Menopause

Around age 40 or 50, your body will slow its production of estrogen and progesterone. Your periods become irregular. This is called premenopause. It may last a few years.

As your levels of estrogen and progesterone drop, your need for insulin may go down. Indeed, this may be a sign that you're starting menopause.

When you have gone a year without a period, menopause is complete. On average, women have their last period around age 50. Some studies show that women with type 1

STATISTICS

Average age at pregnancy for women with type 1 diabetes is 26.

Several clinical studies of women with type 1 diabetes who maintained good blood glucose control before conception and during pregnancy found that the rate of perinatal mortality (death of the infant within 28 days of live birth) was not higher than in the general population.

In one study, women who began intensive diabetes care before becoming pregnant had birth defects in only 1% of their offspring, compared with 10% of offspring of women who began intensive diabetes care after conception.

Women with preexisting diabetic retinopathy are at increased risk of developing advanced stages during gestation. Laser photocoagulation therapy before pregnancy can reduce the chance that advanced diabetes retinopathy will worsen during pregnancy.

diabetes reach menopause up to nine years earlier.

When menopause is complete, if you aren't on hormone replacement therapy, you may find you need up to 20 percent less insulin than you needed before menopause.

Sex

Sex should be as pleasurable for you as for any woman. Diabetes can create a few problems, but all are treatable. Like so many aspects of your health, your sex life can be improved by good blood glucose control.

The fatigue that comes with high blood glucose levels can decrease your desire for sex. High blood glucose levels can also increase your chances of developing vaginal infections, such as recurrent yeast infections. Vaginal infections can make intercourse less desirable.

Sex, like other forms of exercise, can lower your blood glucose levels. Women who wear insulin pumps usually remove them during sex and don't miss the insulin at all. If you use injections, consider decreasing your presex dose or eat a little extra food. Self-monitoring will tell you how your body reacts to sexual excitement.

The most common sexual complaint of women with diabetes is decreased vaginal lubrication leading to painful intercourse. Try an over-the-counter "personal lubricant." In women past menopause, this problem is sometimes treated with estrogen.

Neuropathy can sometimes cause the nerves that supply the genital area to lose feeling. Reaching and maintaining good blood glucose control may help counteract this. You may also want to try vibrators or other forms of stimulation around the clitoris.

If neuropathy has affected your bladder to the extent that you involuntarily urinate during intercourse or orgasm, urinate before and after sex. This is also a good rule of thumb to prevent urinary tract infections.

If you're on dialysis for end-stage renal disease, you may produce large amounts of the hormone prolactin, which decreases sexual desire. Be sure to discuss this with your kidney specialist or doctor.

Birth Control

Imagine this: An unplanned pregnancy. Depending on your circumstances, this might be "not-what-I planned-but-not-terrible" or "terrible."

Now imagine this: An unplanned pregnancy and the birth of an infant with a heart problem, or spina bifida, or kidney problems, a baby who requires several surgeries or hospitalizations. Having diabetes means you have to be extra careful to control your blood glucose to help avoid any problems.

A mother whose blood glucose levels are in the normal, nondiabetic, range during pregnancy, **starting at conception**, will probably have a healthy baby. She has about the same chance of having a baby with a birth defect as a woman who doesn't have diabetes. The rate of birth defects, as well as miscarriage, goes up as blood glucose levels go up.

Many women do achieve near-normal blood glucose levels when they know they're doing it for the health of their babies. But very few people with diabetes walk around in their everyday life with blood glucose levels in the normal range. So effective birth control is hugely important for women and teens who have diabetes.

"I've never been so scared in my life. I thought, I'm pregnant and now it's too late. Something could be wrong and I have to wait eight more months to see if the baby is okay."

—Lee Edwards, whose A1C was 9% when she found out she was four weeks pregnant

---

Your options for birth control are about the same as any woman's. The pill, a diaphragm plus spermicidal jelly, and condom plus spermicidal foam are all good ways to prevent pregnancy. Sterilization is a choice if you want to prevent pregnancy from ever occurring.

An intrauterine device is very effective, but because there is a chance of infection, some doctors don't recommend IUDs for women with diabetes.

Hormone-based methods include Norplant (implanted contraceptive), Depo-Provera (injected contraceptive), and the pill (oral contraceptive). Before prescribing one of these methods, your doctor will consider your health history and whether you have any diabetes complications. If you choose a hormone-based method, be aware that it might affect your blood glucose levels. Your insulin plan may need an adjustment. Check your blood glucose more often when you first start using the method.

Consider doubling up on birth control. For example if you use a diaphragm, which can have a failure rate of 18%, have your partner use a condom. This gives you even more protection from pregnancy and some protection from sexually transmitted diseases, including AIDS.

You can at least double up during your fertile times. You can learn how to tell which days during your cycle you're most likely to get pregnant by monitoring your temperature and the look and feel of your cervical mucus.

Before You Get Pregnant

For the best chance of a successful pregnancy, you need excellent diabetes control both before and during pregnancy. Your baby's organs are formed during the first six to eight weeks after conception. It's critical to have normal blood glucose levels at this time to prevent birth defects. After this time, good glucose control prevents extra glucose from making the baby grow too large.

Birth defects occur in 6% to 12% of the infants of women with diabetes as compared with 2% to 3% of babies of nondiabetic women. In addition, women with diabetes are more likely to have stillbirths and infants with other health problems. These risks can be greatly lowered (although not completely removed) with normal blood glucose levels and good care both before you conceive and during your pregnancy and delivery.

"My first concern was getting pregnant. That is completely the wrong attitude to take. I should have been more concerned about my blood sugars."

—Kim Wilcox

Plan your pregnancy. Start three to six months before you try to conceive. You'll likely need a change in your insulin plan to get the near-normal glucose levels you want for conception. You don't want to be getting used to an insulin pump or learning carbohydrate counting when you conceive. You want your new diabetes plan to be second nature by then.

Blood Glucose Goals At Conception and During Pregnancy

	If your meter tests plasma (mg/dl)	If your meter tests whole blood (mg/dl)
Before meals	80–110	70–100
2 hours after meals	less than 155	less than 140

You also want your A1C in the normal range. Normal range depends on which test is done. A common normal range is 4–6%

Your Medical Team

The ideal health care team for your pregnancy includes

■ a doctor who is a specialist in diabetes
■ an obstetrician with experience in high-risk pregnancies
■ a dietitian
■ a diabetes educator

■ a pediatrician interested in the care of infants of mothers with diabetes

Prepregnancy Exam

You need to get a thorough physical exam by your doctor before you become pregnant. Your doctor will be looking for any health problems that could endanger your health or your baby's. This includes high blood pressure, heart disease, kidney disease, and eye disease. All of these problems should be treated before you become pregnant. Pregnancy can sometimes make them worse. Or they can lead to other problems, such as stroke or heart attack.

If you've had diabetes for more than 10 years and you have other risk factors for heart disease, your doctor may want you to have an electrocardiogram.

Your doctor should look for signs of damage to nerves (neuropathy) that control things such as heart rate and blood vessel opening and narrowing. This diabetes complication can affect how your heart and blood pressure will react to the physical stress of pregnancy.

Gastroparesis results from neuropathy that affects your stomach. Tell your doctor if you have nausea, vomiting, or diarrhea.

Your prepregnancy exam should include your kidneys. In some women, kidney disease may get worse during pregnancy. If you have impaired kidney function, you should know pregnancy may be more difficult for you to manage and you may be troubled by edema (swelling) and high blood pressure.

An eye doctor should examine your retinas through dilated pupils to look for damage due to diabetes (retinopathy). Eye disease should be treated before you become pregnant. Diabetic retinopathy may develop or get worse during pregnancy. It can be treated during pregnancy, so continue to have eye exams during pregnancy. Retinopathy tends to return to its prepregnancy status after delivery.

In addition, your doctor should take a blood sample to measure your thyroid function and to measure your A1C, which shows your overall glucose control.

If you smoke, quit.

Meal Planning

Meal planning will take on a high priority. It's worth it to pay a special visit to your dietitian to get help making dietary changes to meet the demands of pregnancy. Your tighter diabetes control plan will affect how you eat. You may need to switch to three meals and three snacks a day. You may want to learn carbohydrate counting to better match your insulin dose with your meal. You may need strategies for dealing with morning sickness.

Breastfeeding

Breast milk is the ideal food for a new baby. And breastfed babies have a lower risk of type 1 diabetes than formula-fed babies. If you haven't considered breastfeeding, gather information during your pregnancy so you can make an informed choice.

13

Your Health Care Team

These days, diabetes care is viewed as a team effort. You, your family and friends, doctors, diabetes educators, dietitians, and other health care professionals are all players on your health care team.

You

You are the captain of your health care team. When you're well-informed, you can take better care of yourself and get better care from your health care team.

Read *Diabetes Forecast,* the member's magazine of the American Diabetes Association (see p. 189), or other diabetes care magazines each month, and you'll be ahead of the curve. In fact, you may have more new information about diabetes treatment than some family doctors.

As team captain, you're responsible for picking the other players on your team. You'll spend time with these professionals writing a treatment plan that suits your unique needs. Your team can help you in the short term, when you have questions about your insulin, get sick, or need to change your diet. They can also help you over the long term, by working to prevent complications of diabetes such as eye disease, heart disease, nerve damage, and kidney disease.

Primary Care Doctor

You'll see your primary care doctor for general check-ups and when you're sick. Your primary care doctor will be in charge of giving the other health care professionals information about your health and diabetes control.

You may want to go to an endocrinologist. Endocrinologists have thoroughly studied diabetes. If you can't find an endocrinologist nearby, look for a family practice doctor or an internist with expertise in caring for people with diabetes.

The American Diabetes Association's Provider Recognition Program, cosponsored by the National Committee for Quality Assurance (NCQA), is a voluntary program for physicians who provide care to people with diabetes. Physicians can achieve Recognition by submitting data that demonstrates they are providing quality diabetes care. For a Recognized physician in your area, call 800-DIABETES (800-342-2383). Via the internet, go to www.diabetes.org/recognition/provider.

But you can't learn all you need to know during a 1-hour visit with your doctor. Diabetes is a complicated disease, and you will gain from the skill of other health professionals working with your primary care physician. Ask your doctor about who he or she would suggest you have on your team. You may have different team members in different locations, so be sure each team member has phone and fax numbers for the rest of the team so that they can communicate about changes in your control or care.

Your Diabetes Educator

Your doctor wants you to monitor your blood glucose and report the results. But who will help you choose a monitor that's best for your needs, teach you how to use it, and what to do with the results? Who will tell you what you should record in your log about exercise and stress?

Your doctor gives you a prescription for glucagon. But who will teach your needle-phobic spouse how to use it?

Who can help you decide whether it would be safe for your child to go on an overnight camping trip? Who will give you a sick-day plan that includes when you should call your doctor? Whom can you go to when you are fed-up with your blood sugars being out of your goal range?

Your diabetes educator. A diabetes educator is a health care professional—nurse, dietitian, pharmacist, exercise specialist, doctor, or social worker—who specializes in the treatment of people with diabetes. The initials CDE (certified diabetes educator) indicate that the person has passed an exam given by the National Certification Board for Diabetes Educators, is experienced at providing diabetes education, and is up-to-date about diabetes care.

Diabetes educators work in many settings: in hospitals, doctor's offices, neighborhood clinics, pharmacies, or in their own office. Anywhere people with diabetes might regularly go you could find a diabetes educator. The American Association of Diabetes Educators can provide local referrals. Call 1-800-832-6874. Via the internet, go to www.aadenet.org and click on Find a Diabetes Educator.

Diabetes educators provide services in different ways. You could take a class where you'll be able to interact with different educators at different times. These educators might include nurses, dietitians, pharmacists, or even doctors. On the other hand, you might prefer one-on-one interaction with just one educator who can focus on your specific needs.

Attending a diabetes education program is a great way to get started. These programs are usually run where there are many members of your team available such as a hospital or clinic but, like diabetes educators, you may find one anywhere there are many people with diabetes. Look for a program that meets the National Standards for Diabetes Self-Management Education Programs. These programs are recognized by the ADA and have at least a registered dietitian (RD) and a registered nurse (RN) who have continuing education and experience in both diabetes and counseling. Find programs in your area by calling 800-DIABETES (800-342-2383). Via the internet go to www.diabetes.org/education/edustate2.

A good diabetes education program will cover all of the following topics:

- **General facts** about diabetes including what causes it
- **Adjusting** psychologically to caring for your diabetes and teaching others
- **Using your family** or friends for support
- **Understanding your eating plan** and the importance of matching your insulin amount to your meal portions
- **Exercising** wisely to manage blood glucose and avoid hypoglycemia
- **Taking medications** such as insulin effectively
- **Balancing** nutrition, exercise, and medication
- **Testing** your blood glucose accurately and recording it properly
- **Dealing with hyperglycemia and hypoglycemia**—their symptoms, causes, and treatments
- **Handling minor illnesses**
- **Preventing or treating long-term complications**
- **Skin, foot, and dental care**
- **Weighing the benefits** and responsibilities of care, avoiding complications, and understanding the impact of smoking and alcohol on diabetes
- **Using the health care system**, including your health care team, to help you take care of your diabetes

■ **Finding community resources** for help with all aspects of diabetes

Your Dietitian

A registered dietitian is a health care professional with training and expertise in the field of food and nutrition. A dietitian helps you understand the role of nutrition in your management plan and helps you develop a meal plan—a crucial component to living well with diabetes.

Look for the initials RD (registered dietitian), which tell you that the dietitian has passed a national credentialing exam. Many states also require a license, so you'll often see the initials LD (licensed dietitian). Some dietitians are also CDEs. The American Dietetic Association (1-800-366-1655, www.eatright.org) can recommend qualified dietitians in your area. Other good sources of recommendations are your primary care doctor, area hospitals, and your local American Diabetes Association affiliate.

An assessment visit generally takes an hour to an hour and a half. Follow-up visits run about 30 minutes or longer, depending on your needs. Follow-up visits allow for sharing further helpful information, progress checks, and adjustments to your meal plan.

Dietitians teach you many useful skills: how to use Exchange Lists for Meal Planning, how to count dietary carbohydrate and make adjustments in your insulin dose, how to read food labels, and how to make healthy food choices when grocery shopping.

Dietitians help you discover a range of nutritional resources, including cookbooks and reference materials, so you can learn how to prepare healthy, delicious, and satisfying meals. They can help you add spice to your life by showing you how to maintain good blood glucose control even when you eat in restaurants, throw a party, or eat a Thanksgiving feast earlier than you normally would eat dinner.

It's a good idea to see a dietitian for a diet assessment every 6 months to a year, or more often if needed. Your meal plan can be adapted to special goals such as weight loss or reducing dietary fat and sodium, and also to your likes and dislikes, work schedule, and lifestyle.

Does your meal plan need a change? If you answer yes to any of the following questions, then it's time your meal plan was brought up-to-date.

- Has your meal plan been reviewed in the last year?
- Is your diabetes or body weight more difficult to control than usual?
- Are you bored with your meals?
- Have you started an exercise program or changed your insulin plan since your last visit with a dietitian?
- Do you want to prevent or have you been diagnosed with high blood pressure, high cholesterol levels, or kidney disease?

Who Pays?

Most states require private insurance policies and managed care plans to include coverage of diabetes self-management training. Contact your American Diabetes Association by phone (1-800-DIABETES) or the Internet (www.diabetes.org) to see if your state has such a law.

If you have Medicare part B (services outside of the hospital), nutrition counseling is a covered service, but you must go to an RD who is a Medicare provider.

If you have health coverage through a large employer, you may or may not be able to get nutrition counseling covered. Call your health plan and ask if they cover this benefit. Ask if you need a referral from your doctor. Health plans often require a written referral to document "medical necessity." Also ask if there are certain dietitians you must go to in order to have your insurer cover the sessions, and how many sessions they cover.

If you don't have a health plan that covers nutrition counseling or no health plan at all, consider paying for it yourself. Your health is worth it. A nutrition counseling session costs $50 to $150. Some dietitians offer a package that includes a number of sessions.

Your Exercise Physiologist

Exercise physiologists can help you select proper exercises, set realistic goals, and stay motivated and disciplined in your exercise routine. They can tailor programs to your health needs. You may want to improve your cardiovascular fitness, lower your blood glucose, lose weight, or develop muscle strength and flexibility. Special exercise programs help you work out even if you are overweight, have been inactive for a long time, or have arthritis. You should have your primary-care physician approve any exercise program you select.

Look for someone with a master's or doctoral degree in exercise physiology or a licensed health care professional with graduate training in this area. You may want someone certified by the American College of Sports Medicine.

Your Mental Health Counselor

Diabetes brings its share of stresses. You may benefit from seeing a therapist, such as a social worker, family therapist, psychologist, or psychiatrist. This person can help you deal with the personal and emotional aspects of diabetes.

A social worker should have a master's degree in social work (MSW), as well as training in individual, group, and family therapy. Social workers can help you cope with many issues relating to diabetes control, from problems in the family or in work situations to locating resources to help with medical or financial needs.

A marriage and family therapist should have a master's degree in a mental health field and added training in individual, family, and marriage therapy. These therapists can help you with personal difficulties in your family, your marriage, or your job.

A clinical psychologist has a master's or doctoral degree in psychology and is trained in individual, group, and family psychology. You might visit a psychologist during a particularly stressful few weeks or months or on a long-term basis to work out more deep-seated problems.

A psychiatrist is a doctor with the medical training to understand how the physical aspects of diabetes can contribute to your psychological health. A psychiatrist can also prescribe medications or hospitalization for emotional problems when needed.

Your Eye Doctor

Ophthalmologists are medical doctors who can treat eye problems both medically and surgically. Retina specialists are ophthalmologists with further training in the diagnosis and treatment of diseases of the retina. Optometrists are trained in examining the eye for certain problems, such as how well your eyes focus. They are not medical doctors and are not able to prescribe medications in some states. Ophthalmologists and optometrists both do dilated eye exams.

You should see an ophthalmologist if you, your family doctor, or your optometrist notice any of the following signs:

- **Spots, "floaters," or cobwebs** in your field of vision; blurred or distorted vision; blind spots; eye pain; persistent redness.
- **Loss of your ability to read** books or traffic signs, or to distinguish familiar objects.
- **Increased pressure within the eye** (a warning sign of glaucoma). Some internal medicine and family doctors and most optometrists test for this.

■ **Any abnormality of the retina.**
Internists, family practitioners, and
optometrists should test for this but
should refer retinal problems to ophthalmologists. Retinopathy, the leaking of
blood vessels that supply the retina, is
the main cause of blindness in people
with diabetes.

Your Podiatrist

People with diabetes can develop poor blood
flow and nerve damage in their feet. Sores,
even small ones, can quickly turn into serious
problems. Your primary care physician may
refer you to a podiatrist. Podiatrists graduate
from a college of podiatry with a Doctor of
Podiatric Medicine (DPM) degree. They have
completed residencies in podiatry and can do
surgery and prescribe medicine.

It's a good idea to see a podiatrist
before you have a problem. The podiatrist
will check the pulses in your feet to see
whether you have good circulation. He or she
will check to see whether you have nerve
damage in your feet (see pp. 139–141).

A foot deformity, such as a hammertoe,
puts you at higher risk of developing a foot
ulcer. Your podiatrist may recommend that
you have surgery to correct the deformity
while you are young and have good circulation in your feet, so you'll heal quickly after
surgery. This can prevent problems in the
future.

Your Pharmacist

You're having a medical problem and the specialist you're seeing wrote you a prescription. Will that medication affect your blood glucose levels? When should you test your blood sugar to find out? Will any of the medications you're taking (including over-the-counter remedies) interact with any of your other medications? Are there any side effects? What should you take for a cold when you have diabetes?

Whom do you ask? Your pharmacist.

Your pharmacist is a valuable resource when working with you and your team. You can help your pharmacist help you by choosing a pharmacist you like and who knows about diabetes. You might even find one who is a CDE or is a Certified Disease Manager (CDM) in diabetes. Ask your doctor or diabetes educator which pharmacy or pharmacist they recommend, and then stick with them. To give you the best service, your pharmacist needs to keep an accurate, up-to-date profile of your medical history, allergies, and medications. If you move from pharmacy to pharmacy, no one pharmacist will have all the information needed to screen your medication regimens.

Ask questions. When you are concerned about possible side effects, when to take your medication, what to do when you miss dose, or how to store your medications, call your pharmacist. They might also be able to refer you to other resources in your area for managing your diabetes.

Your Dentist

Just like people, bacteria love sweets. When you have high glucose levels, your saliva makes your mouth a home for the bacteria that cause gum infection. And diabetes can also make it harder for your mouth to fight infections once they start.

To dodge gum disease, get your teeth cleaned at your dentist's every 6 months. Tell the dentist you have diabetes, and ask the dentist or dental hygienist to check your brushing and flossing technique. Beyond regular visits, you should call the dentist if you notice any signs of gum disease, such as bleeding when you floss, or gums that are puffy or sore.

A WINTER EVENING'S DISCOURSE

A few years ago, I took a faculty position at a small, liberal arts college. When I traded in my counselor's hat for a career in teaching, I was looking forward to those deep philosophical discussions that professors seem to have with anyone within earshot.

My wife, Tammi, and I had always enjoyed such discussions, but our time at home was becoming increasingly consumed with typical family concerns: what to have for dinner, whether or not to paint the bathroom, and how our first-grader, Joshua, did in school that day. I was pleasantly surprised one evening last winter when the opportunity for a thought-provoking talk presented itself.

We settled on spaghetti for dinner, white paint for the bathroom, and heard the latest of Joshua's school adventures. Then the topic turned to whether or not we believed my diabetes would one day be cured.

I don't recall how we stumbled upon this subject, but it was certainly one that challenged both Tammi and me. On the one hand, it was a mental exercise perfectly suited to my need for a philosophical debate. On the other hand, it was an emotional can of worms, setting us up for the thrill of the possibility of a cure, and gloom at the thought that it might not happen in my lifetime.

We were surprised to find how difficult it was to even imagine something so far outside our normal frame of reference.

It was more complex than the fancy of going on a long mountain hike without backup food. To understand what it really feels like to live without diabetes involved a complete reconceptualization of almost every aspect of day-to-day existence.

I grew up with diabetes; it's an intimate part of my life. I used it to manipulate my parents during adolescence. I knew it was there when I registered for the draft during the Vietnam war. It qualified me for scholarship money to attend college. It was with me when I met Tammi, and it has been part of both of our lives ever since.

In graduate school, the psychological aspects of diabetes filled my research papers, and my dissertation focused on job performance and diabetes. I established a private counseling practice in diabetes management and have continued to be interested in diabetes issues, especially those involving the Americans With Disabilities Act.

I even have diabetes in my dreams.

As Tammi and I talked, I tried remembering back more than 30 years, to the 10 years of my life before I was diagnosed with diabetes. Although I could recall selected events, I couldn't remember what it really felt like to be free of injections, blood sugar tests, and meal planning.

Tammi and I decided that this all goes to show how much I've accepted my diabetes. However, neither of us were sure we accepted that I will always have diabetes. At this point, we uncovered the real issue of our discussion: our ongoing struggle to balance acceptance with the right amount of hope.

I told Tammi about one very clear memory from childhood. It was a statement made by the physician who diagnosed my diabetes. He told me there would be a "cure" within five years. Despite his best intentions, he gave my parents and me a great deal of false hope.

Yet even with that tough lesson learned, I often fall victim to press releases announcing the most recent "cure for diabetes." These are frequently used in the media as a tease to watch the 10 o'clock news or listen to an upcoming radio report. In addition, research facilities can benefit financially by raising hopes.

I am all for reporting the latest research and raising the money to fund it. However, I resent the letdown that comes when I realize it will be years, at best, before these "cures" are actually available.

At the same time, I must admit that not all my hopes come from external sources. Sometimes, I simply give in to the need to feel like there is an end in sight. This temporary reprieve is a pleasant escape, and by keeping my spirits up, it helps me successfully manage my diabetes.

Tammi and I could not say for sure if we will ever know life without diabetes, but we did realize the value of that dream. So we ended our discussion with a toast: To just the right amount of hoping.

David Greene
Diabetes Forecast
December 1997

14

How To . . .

How to Self-Monitor Your Blood Glucose

Follow your meter manufacturer's instructions for best results. If you have problems, there should be a toll-free number in the printed instructions or on the meter that you can call for help.

Equipment:

- **Lancet**
- **Fresh test strip**
- **Blood glucose meter**
  1. Wash your hands and dry them thoroughly. Soap, lotion, or food on your hands can cause incorrect test results. It's also not a good idea to use alcohol since alcohol can dry out your fingers.
  2. Place a lancet in your lancet device and a strip in your meter according to the manufacturer's instructions.

3. Puncture the skin as recommended by the meter manufacturer, such as a finger, forearm, or thigh depending on which meter you use. If you use your fingers, it's more comfortable to use the side of your finger than the tip. It's also usually easier to get blood there.

4. Squeeze out a drop of blood. If you start at your palm and squeeze up to the tip you shouldn't have trouble getting a drop.

5. Place the blood drop on the pad of a test strip or touch the strip to the drop of blood depending on which type of strip you are using. Your meter will start counting down when the appropriate amount of blood is applied. If the meter doesn't start, use a fresh strip and try again using a larger drop of blood.

6. Dispose of the lancet safely by replacing the cap or placing it in an appropriate "sharps" container.

7. Record your numbers.

How to Test for Ketones in Your Urine

Check for ketones when:

■ Several blood glucose tests in a day are 240 mg/dl or higher, or
■ You are sick or feel queasy
   1. Dip a ketone test strip in a urine sample or pass it through the stream of urine.

2. Time the test according to the directions on the package (10 seconds to 2 minutes, depending on the brand).
3. There will be a color change if ketones are present. Compare color to package color chart.
4. Record the results.

How to Prepare an Insulin Injection

Equipment:

▓ **Sterile syringe.** Use the smallest size syringe and needle for your dose and body type. Ask your doctor, diabetes educator, or pharmacist which is best for you.

▓ **Bottle of insulin**

▓ **Alcohol swab**, if desired, to clean the injection site or the insulin bottle

1. Wash hands.
2. Choose injection site.
3. Roll the bottle of insulin between your hands. (Clear insulins don't need to be rolled.) Don't shake it, because this makes air bubbles in the insulin. Air bubbles interfere with correct measurement of the units of insulin.
4. Wipe the top of the bottle with an alcohol swab, then let the alcohol dry completely.
5. Holding the syringe with the needle pointing up, draw air into it by pulling down on the plunger to the amount that matches your insulin dose.

6. Remove the cap from the needle. Hold the insulin bottle steady on a table top, and push the needle straight down into the rubber top on the bottle. Push down on the plunger to inject the air into the insulin bottle.

7. Leave the needle in the bottle and the plunger pushed all the way in while you pick up the bottle and turn it upside down. The point of the needle should be covered by the insulin.

8. Pull the correct amount of insulin into the syringe by pulling back slowly on the plunger.

9. Check for air bubbles on the inside of the syringe. If you see air bubbles and have not mixed different insulins in the same syringe, keep the bottle upside down and push the plunger up so the insulin goes back into the bottle.

10. Pull down on the plunger to refill the syringe. If necessary, empty and refill until all air bubbles in the syringe are gone.

11. Remove the needle from the bottle after checking again that you have the correct dose.

12. If you need to set the syringe down before giving your injection, recap and lay it on its side. Make sure the needle doesn't touch anything.

How to Mix Insulins

Equipment:

- **Sterile disposable syringe**, the correct size for the total units of insulin
- **Bottles of each type of insulin** you are going to use. NOTE: Not all insulins can be mixed together (pp. 15–16). Always check with your doctor, diabetes educator, or pharmacist before mixing insulins.
- **Alcohol swab**, if desired, to clean the injection site or the insulin bottle
    1. Be sure of the amount of each insulin and the total units you want. To find the total units, add the units of rapid-acting insulin to the units of long-acting insulin.
    2. Wash your hands.
    3. Mix the cloudy insulin by rolling the bottle of insulin between your hands.
    4. Draw air into the syringe equal to the amount of intermediate- or long-acting dose (cloudy).
    5. With the bottle upright on a table, inject the air into that bottle. Take out the needle without removing any insulin.
    6. Draw air into the syringe equal to the dose of rapid- or short-acting insulin and inject the air into the upright bottle of rapid-acting insulin.
    7. With the needle still in the rapid-acting insulin bottle, turn it upside down so that insulin covers the top of the needle.

8. Pull the correct amount of insulin into the syringe by pulling back on the plunger. If necessary, empty and refill until all air bubbles in the syringe are gone. Remove the syringe.

9. With the bottle of intermediate- or long-acting insulin held upside down, insert the syringe. (You have already injected the right amount of air into this bottle.)

10. Slowly pull the plunger to draw in the right dosage of intermediate- or long-acting insulin. Remember you need to draw back to the total units of the short- plus intermediate- or long-acting insulins.

11. Do not return any extra insulin back to this bottle. It's now a mixture. Double check for the correct total amount of insulin. If you over-drew, discard the syringe and contents and start over.

12. Take the needle out of the bottle, recap, and lay the syringe carefully on a table without it touching anything until you use it.

How to Store Mixed Insulins

1. Check with the manufacturer, your diabetes educator, or your pharmacist about how long you can store mixed insulins. Some mixtures need to be used right after they're mixed.

2. Keep the prefilled syringes capped.

3. Before injection, pull back on the plunger a little and tip the syringe back and forth a few times to remix the insulin. Carefully push the plunger back to its original position, pushing air out of the syringe but not insulin.

How to Inject Insulin

Equipment:

■ **Prepared filled sterile syringe**
■ **Alcohol swab** to wipe the injection site if desired

1. Choose an injection site with fatty tissue, such as the backs of the arms, the top and outside of the thighs, the abdomen except for a 1-inch square around the belly button, or the buttocks. Do not inject into or close to any scars. Make sure the site and your hands are clean.

2. Use the correct needle for your body type to eliminate the need for pinching the skin. Inject straight in if you have a normal amount of fatty tissue.

3. Push the needle through the skin. Try to avoid rocking the syringe. Keeping the needle straight makes the injection more comfortable.

4. Slowly (a count of 3–5 is usually sufficient) push the plunger in to inject the insulin.

5. Wait a few seconds to allow all the insulin to be delivered then pull the needle straight out.

6. Write down how much insulin you injected, the time of day, and the site you chose.

If You Reuse Your Syringe

Disposable syringes were designed for one use only and manufacturers don't recommend reuse. Each time you use a needle it gets duller.

1. Carefully recap the syringe when you aren't using it.
2. Don't let the needle touch anything but clean skin and your insulin bottle stopper. If it touches anything else, don't reuse it.
3. Store the used syringe at room temperature.
4. There will always be a tiny, even invisible, amount of insulin left in the syringe and needle. So use one syringe with just one type of insulin to avoiding mixing insulins. For this reason, reusing syringes in which you have mixed insulins is not recommended.
5. Do not reuse a needle that is bent or dull.
6. Don't wipe your needle with alcohol. This removes some of the coating that makes the needle go more smoothly into your skin.
7. When you're finished with a syringe, dispose of it properly according to the laws in your area. Contact the city or county sanitation department for information.

What to Teach Others About Mixing and Injecting Glucagon

Glucagon is not stable as a liquid, so it's stored unmixed. Someone needs to mix it and then inject it. Glucagon is available by prescription, and it comes two ways:

- a bottle of powdered glucagon and a syringe filled with diluting fluid (more convenient), or
- a bottle of powdered glucagon and a bottle of diluting fluid (less convenient but also less expensive).

  1. Remove the flip-off seal from the bottle of glucagon.
  2. Fill a syringe with the diluting fluid (or use the prefilled syringe).
  3. Inject ALL the diluting fluid into the bottle of glucagon.
  4. Remove the syringe. Shake the bottle gently until the solution is clear.
  5. Using the same syringe, withdraw all of the solution from the bottle. **(If the dose is for a child under age 6, use only 1/2 of the solution.)**
  6. Inject glucagon in the same way and in the same parts of the body that you inject insulin.
  7. The person may feel nauseated or vomit. Keep the head elevated and tilted to the side.
  8. When the person is able to drink or eat (should be within 2 to 10 minutes), offer sips of juice or other form of sugar. Then offer food.

9. Check blood glucose.
10. When the episode is over, remember to let your doctor know you had a severe low blood sugar.

If glucagon does not revive the person, or if glucagon is not available, call 911.

15

Diabetes Resources

Your American Diabetes Association

The American Diabetes Association (ADA) is the nation's leading nonprofit health organization providing diabetes research, information, and advocacy. Founded in 1940, the American Diabetes Association conducts programs in all 50 states and the District of Columbia, reaching more than 800 communities.

The mission of ADA is to prevent and cure diabetes and to improve the lives of all people affected by diabetes. To fulfill this mission, the American Diabetes Association funds research; publishes scientific findings; provides information and other services to people with diabetes, their families, health care professionals, and the public; and advocates for scientific research and for the rights of people with diabetes.

The moving force behind our work is a network of more than one million volunteers, including a membership of 390,000 diabetes patients and their families, and a professional society of more than 20,000 researchers and health care providers.

1-800-DIABETES

The National Call Center provides diabetes information and referral for callers nationwide through our toll-free 800 number. The Call Center responds to approximately 350,000 inquiries each year. Callers can get information on:

■ **Diabetes education classes**
■ **Year-round youth programs**
■ **Counseling and support groups**
■ **Advocacy services**
■ **Information and referral services**

diabetes.org

The American Diabetes Association's Web site, diabetes.org, is the largest interactive diabetes site on the Internet. On the site, people can find information about diabetes and living with the disease, register for special events, buy books, make a donation, tour an interactive grocery store, read journal abstracts, and much more. With more than 206 million hits recorded in fiscal year 2001, the Web site remains a popular medium to reach the Association's constituencies.

You can go to the Web bookstore directly at store.diabetes.org (no www) or call 1-800-232-6733 to order books.

Advocacy

The American Diabetes Association takes tough positions on issues important to people with diabetes. Our advocacy activities include:

■ Working to increase federal funding for diabetes research and programs
■ Working to improve insurance coverage and healthcare for people with diabetes
■ Working to end discrimination against people with diabetes

Professional Services

The Association provides educational and other informative materials and programs for health care professionals to improve care for people with diabetes. These include:

■ Annual Scientific Sessions, the world's largest diabetes conference
■ Medical care guidelines and recommendations
■ Diabetes patient education program accreditation
■ Provider Recognition Program (see below)

■ The journals *Diabetes*, *Diabetes Care*, *Diabetes Spectrum*, and *Clinical Diabetes*, and a comprehensive library of medical management guides

Program Services
The Diabetes Assistance and Resources Program (DAR)

DAR, which means "to give" in Spanish, provides valuable information in English and Spanish to the Latino/Hispanic community. The goal of the DAR program is to increase awareness about the seriousness of diabetes and the importance of prevention and control.

African American Program

The African American Program's goal is to increase awareness about the seriousness of diabetes in the community and importance of early diagnosis and treatment. The program includes fun and informative church and community-based activities such as "Diabetes Sunday" and "Get Up and Move."

Awakening the Spirit: Pathways to Diabetes Prevention and Control

Awakening the Spirit disseminates critical messages about the seriousness of diabetes to the Native American community, including American Indians, Alaska Natives, and Native Hawaiians. The program stresses the importance of choosing a healthy lifestyle for oneself and the generations that will follow.

Public Awareness Activities
American Diabetes Month

American Diabetes Month is the Association's annual, month-long public awareness activity held each November for people with diabetes and their families. The goal is to raise awareness about serious and often preventable diabetes complications. A variety of events and educational activities are included in this awareness effort.

American Diabetes Alert

The American Diabetes Alert is conducted annually on the fourth Tuesday in March to raise awareness about the seriousness of diabetes and its risk factors. The centerpiece of the Alert is the diabetes risk test, which is widely distributed and promoted through community activities and national and local media.

Publications

The Association is the world's foremost publisher in the field of diabetes literature including:

- *Diabetes Forecast*, a monthly magazine to help people with diabetes live fuller, healthier lives
- A comprehensive library of cookbooks and meal-planning guides, and food-exchange lists
- Books, brochures, and pamphlets on every aspect of living with diabetes

Recognized Providers

The American Diabetes Association's Provider Recognition Program, cosponsored by the National Committee for Quality Assurance (NCQA), is a voluntary program for physicians who provide care to people with diabetes. Physicians can achieve Recognition by submitting data that demonstrates they are providing quality diabetes care. Find a Recognized physician in your area by checking www.diabetes.org/recognition/provider or calling 1-800-DIABETES.

For a diabetes education program that meets the National Standards for Diabetes Self-Management Education Programs and are recognized by the ADA, go to www.diabetes.org/education/edustate2 or call 1-800-DIABETES.

Research

To date, the Association has invested more than $200 million in diabetes research throughout the nation. The Association raises these critical funds through many vehicles, including its Research Foundation, special events, direct mail campaigns, and corporate partners. Recent advances in research include:

- More precise methods to identify people who are at risk for diabetes and potential treatments to prevent the onset of the disease
- Improved techniques for islet cell transplantation
- Laser therapy to prevent diabetes-related blindness

- Better understanding of the importance of nutrition and psychosocial factors in diabetes treatment
- Researchers moving ever-closer to identifying the "diabetes genes"

Youth Programs (Wizdom)
www.diabetes.org/wizdom
The new American Diabetes Association Wizdom program provides a kit of "wit and wisdom" for newly diagnosed youth with diabetes and their families and features a fun and educational Web site. The program emphasizes teaching kids and families to "juggle" the three main aspects of diabetes—food, exercise, and insulin—to maintain good diabetes control.

Camps for Children with Diabetes
www.diabetes.org/wizdom/camps.asp
Join in the summer camp fun! This Web site gives a state-by-state listing of camps for children with diabetes. Both resident and day camps are offered. Camps are classified as either operated by the American Diabetes Association, or marketed and financially supported by the Association. Camps on this site are accredited by the American Camping Association or have met basic safety standards. You can learn more about diabetes camp in a new book by ADA, *Getting the Most Out of Diabetes Camp: A Guidebook for Parents and Kids*, 2002, $14.95.

For the Visually Challenged

American Printing House for the Blind
1839 Frankfort Avenue
P.O. Box 6085
Louisville, KY 40206-0085
502-895-2405
502-899-2274 (fax)
800-223-1839
e-mail: info@aph.org
Web site: www.aph.org
Concerned with the publication of literature in all media
(Braille, large type, recorded) and manufacture of
educational aids. Newsletter provides information on new
products.

**National Association for Visually Handicapped
(NAVH)**
22 West 21st Street
New York, NY 10010
212-889-3141
Web site: www.navh.org

or

**NAVH San Francisco regional office
(for states west of the Mississippi)**
3201 Balboa Street
San Francisco, CA 94121
415-221-3201
A list of low-vision facilities is available by state. Visual aid
counseling and visual aids, peer support groups, and more
intensive counseling are offered at both offices. Some
counseling is done by mail or phone. Maintains a large-print
loan library.

National Federation of the Blind
1800 Johnson Street
Baltimore, MD 21230
410-659-9314 (for general information)
800-638-7518 (for job opportunities for the blind)
Web site: http://www.nfb.org
Membership organization providing information,
networking, and resources through 52 affiliates in all states,
the District of Columbia, and Puerto Rico. Some aids and
appliances available through national headquarters. The
Diabetics Division publishes a free quarterly newsletter,
Voice of the Diabetic, in print or on cassette.

National Library Service (NLS) for the Blind and Physically Handicapped
Library of Congress
1291 Taylor Street NW
Washington, DC 20542
202-707-5100
202-707-0744 (TDD)
800-424-8567 (to speak with a reference person)
800-424-9100 (to leave a message)
e-mail: nls@loc.gov
Web site: http://www.loc.gov/nls/
Encore, a monthly magazine on flexible disk (record), includes articles from *Diabetes Forecast*. It is available on request through the NLS program to individuals registered with the talking book program.

Recording for the Blind & Dyslexic (RFBD)
20 Roszel Road
Princeton, NJ 08540
609-452-0606
609-987-8116 (fax)
800-221-4792 (weekdays 8:30–4:45 EST)
Web site: http://www.rfbd.org
Library for people with print disabilities. Provides educational materials in recorded and computerized form; 80,000 titles on cassette. Registration fee of $50.00 includes loan of cassettes for up to a year.

For Finding Quality Health Care

American Association for Marriage and Family Therapy
112 S. Alfred Street
Alexandria, VA 22314
703-838-9808
e-mail: memberservice@aamft.org
Web site: http://www.aamft.org
For marriage and family therapists in your area, send a self-addressed, stamped envelope to the attention of Mr. Johnson.

American Association of Diabetes Educators
100 W. Monroe Street, Suite 400
Chicago, IL 60603
312-424-2426
312-424-2427
800-832-6874 (referral line)
Web site: http://www.aadenet.org
Referral to a local diabetes educator.

American Association of Sex Educators, Counselors, and Therapists

P.O. Box 238
Mount Vernon, IA 52314-0238
For a list of certified sex therapists and counselors in your
state, send a self-addressed, stamped, business-size envelope
(you may request lists from more than one state).

American Board of Medical Specialties

47 Perimeter Center East, Suite 500
Atlanta, GA 30346
866-275-2267
866-ASKABMS
Web site: http://www.abms.org
Record of physicians certified by 24 medical specialty boards.
Only certification status of physician is available to callers.
Directories of certified physicians organized by city of
medical practice and alphabetically by physician names are
available in many libraries.

American Board of Podiatric Surgery

3330 Mission Street
San Francisco, CA 94110
415-826-3200
415-826-4640 (fax)
e-mail: info@abps.org
Web site: http://www.abps.org
Referral to a local board-certified podiatrist.

The American Dietetic Association

216 West Jackson Boulevard, Suite 800
Chicago, IL 60606
312-899-0040
312-899-1979 (fax)
800-366-1655 Consumer Nutrition Hot Line; 9–4 CST, M–F
only
Web site: http://www.eatright.org
Information, guidance, and referral to a local dietitian.

American Medical Association

515 North State Street
Chicago, IL 60610
312-464-4818
Web site: http://www.ama–assn.org
Referral to your county or state medical society, which may
be able to refer you to a local physician.

American Optometric Association
243 N. Lindbergh Boulevard
St. Louis, MO 63141
314-991-4100
314-991-4101 (fax)
Web site: http://www.aoanet.org
Referral to your state optometric association for referral to a
local optometrist.

American Psychiatric Association
1400 K Street NW
Washington, DC 20005
202-682-6000
202-682-6114 (fax)
888-357-7924
e-mail: apa@psych.org
Web site: http://www.psych.org
Referral to your state psychiatric association for referral to a
local psychiatrist.

American Psychological Association
750 First Street NE
Washington, DC 20002-4242
202-336-5500 (main number)
202-336-5700 (public affairs)
202-436-5800 (professional practice)
800-374-2721
Web site: http://www.apa.org
Referral to your state psychological association for referral
to a local psychologist.

National Association of Social Workers
750 First Street NE, Suite 700
Washington, DC 20002-4247
202-408-8600
800-638-8799
Web site: http://www.naswdc.org
Referral to your state chapter of NASW for referral to a
local social worker.

Pedorthic Footwear Association
7150 Columbia Gateway Drive, Suite G
Columbia, MD 21046
410-381-7278
410-381-1167 (fax)
800-673-8447
Web site: http://www.pedorthics.org
Referral to a local certified pedorthist (a person trained in
fitting prescription footwear).

For Miscellaneous Health Information

American Academy of Ophthalmology
Customer Service Department
P.O. Box 7424
San Francisco, CA 94120-7424
415-561-8500
415-561-8533 (fax)
Web site: http://www.aao.org
For brochures on eye care and eye diseases, send a self-addressed, stamped envelope.

American Heart Association
7272 Greenville Avenue
Dallas, TX 75231
800-242-8721
Web site: http://www.americanheart.org
For referral to local affiliate's *Heartline*, which provides information on cardiovascular health and disease prevention.

Medic Alert Foundation
P.O. Box 1009
Turlock, CA 95381-1009
209-668-3331
209-669-2495 (fax)
800-432-5378
Web site: http://www.medicalert.org
To order a medical I.D. bracelet.

National Chronic Pain Outreach Association
P.O. Box 274
Millboro, VA 24460
540-862-9437
540-862-9485 (fax)
e-mail: ncpoa@cfw.com
To learn more about chronic pain and how to deal with it.

National Kidney Foundation
30 E. 33rd Street
New York, NY 10016
212-889-2210
212-689-9261 (fax)
800-622-9010
e-mail: info@kidney.org
Web site: http://www.kidney.org
For donor cards and information about kidney disease and transplants.

United Network for Organ Sharing
1100 Boulders Parkway, Suite 500
P.O. Box 13770
Richmond, VA 23225-8770
804-330-8602 (communications)
800-355-SHARE (for information on becoming a donor)
800-24-DONOR
Web site: http://www.unos.org
For information about organ transplants and a list of organ
transplant centers in the U.S.

For Travelers
**International Association for Medical Assistance
to Travelers**
417 Center Street
Lewiston, NY 14092
716-754-4883
519-836-3412 (fax)
Web site: http://www.iamat.org
For a list of doctors in foreign countries who speak English
and who received postgraduate training in North America or
Great Britain.

International Diabetes Federation
40 Washington Street
B–1050 Brussels, Belgium
Web site: http://www.idf.org
For a list of International Diabetes Federation groups that
can offer assistance when you're traveling.

For Exercisers
American College of Sports Medicine
P.O. Box 1440
Indianapolis, IN 46206-1440
317-637-9200
317-634-7817 (fax)
Web site: http://www.acsm.org
For information about health and fitness.

International Diabetic Athletes Association
1647 W. Bethany Home Road, #B
Phoenix, AZ 85015-2507
800-898-IDAA
e-mail: idaa@getnet.com
For people with diabetes and for health care professionals
interested in exercise and fitness at all levels. Newsletter.

For People Over 50
National Council on the Aging
409 3rd Street SW, Suite 200
Washington, DC 20024
202-479-1200
202-479-0735 (fax)
800-424-9046
Web site: http://www.ncoa.org
Advocacy group concerned with developing and
implementing high standards of care for the elderly. Referral
to local agencies concerned with the elderly.

For Equal Employment Information
American Bar Association
Commission on Mental and Physical Disability Law
740 15th Street NW
Washington, DC 20005-1009
202-662-1570
202-662-1032 (fax)
202-662-1012 (TTY)
e-mail: cmpdl@abanet.org
Web site: http://www.abanet.org/disability
Provides information and technical assistance on all aspects
of disability law.

Disability Rights Education and Defense Fund, Inc.
2212 6th Street
Berkeley, CA 94710
510-644-2555 (voice/TDD)
510-841-8645 (fax)
800-466-4232 (voice/TDD)
e-mail: dredfca@dredf.org
Web site: http://www.dredf.org
Provides technical assistance and information to employers
and individuals with disabilities on disability rights
legislation and policies. Assists with legal representation.

Equal Employment Opportunity Commission
1801 L Street NW
Washington, DC 20507
For technical assistance and filing a charge:
202-663-4900
202-663-4912 (fax)
202-663-4494 (TTY)
800-669-4000 (connects to nearest local EEOC office)
800-669-3362 (for publications)
800-669-6820 (TDD)
Web site: http://www.eeoc.gov

**National Information Center for Children
and Youth With Disabilities**
P.O. Box 1492
Washington, DC 20013-1492
202-884-8200 (voice and TTY)
202-884-8441 (fax)
800-695-0285 (voice and TTY)
Web site: http://www.nichcy.org
Provides technical assistance and information on disabilities
and disability-related issues.

For Health Insurance Information
AARP health insurance
800-523-5800
800-523-7773 (TTY)
Web site: http://www.aarp.org
The AARP administers 10 health insurance plans. For some
plans, individuals with diabetes or other chronic illnesses
are eligible within 6 months after enrolling in Medicare
Part B. For other plans, a 3-month waiting period is required
for those with conditions preexistent in the 6 months
preceding the effective date of the insurance, if not replacing
previous coverage.

Medicare Hot Line
800-MEDICARE
U.S. Department of Health and Human Services
Centers for Medicine and Medicaid Services
6325 Security Boulevard
Baltimore, MD 21207
Web site: http://www.medicare.gov
For information and various publications about Medicare.

Social Security Administration
800-772-1213
Web site: http://www.ssa.gov
For information and various publications about Medicare.

Helpful Websites
www.diabetes.org (ADA website)

www.niddk.nih.gov/health/diabetes/diabetes.htm
(NIH/NIDDK government website)

www.childrenwithdiabetes.com (created by a father;
offers many chat rooms and answers to more than
3,000 questions on-line)

www.diabetesmonitor.com (supplies information on upcoming medications and research, plus a mentor section)

www.mendosa.com/diabetes.htm (a diabetes directory)

www.diabetes.com (lots of news from medical journals)

You can also subscribe to the following list servers (groups of people who share information about a topic):

listserv@lehigh.edu. To subscribe, send an e-mail to the list serve. In the message box write the words "subscribe diabetic your name" (write your name here).

majordomo@world.std.com. To subscribe, send an e-mail to the list serve. In the message box write the words "subscribe diabetes."

ADA Division Offices
Northeastern Division
149 Madison Avenue, 8th Floor
New York, NY 10016
212-725-4925
Joyce Waite, Vice President

Connecticut, Delaware, D.C., Maine, Maryland, Massachusetts, New Jersey, New York, New Hampshire, Northern Virginia, Pennsylvania, Vermont, and Rhode Island

Mountain/Pacific Division
2480 West 26th Avenue, Suite 120B
Denver, CO 80211
720-855-1102
Mike Van Abel, Vice President

Alaska, Arizona, Colorado, Hawaii, Idaho, Montana, New Mexico, Oregon, Utah, Washington, Wyoming

North Central Division
2323 North Mayfair Rd. #502
Wauwatosa, WI 53226
414-778-5500
Lew Bartfield, Vice President

Iowa, Illinois, Indiana, Michigan, Minnesota,
Nebraska, North Dakota, Ohio, South Dakota,
Wisconsin, West Virginia

South Central Division
4425 West Airport Freeway, Suite 130
Irving, TX 75062
972-255-6900
Quin Neal, Vice President

Arkansas, Kansas, Louisiana, Mississippi, Missouri,
Oklahoma, Texas

South Coastal Division
1101 North Lake Destiny Road, Suite 415
Maitland, Florida 32751
407-660-1926
Nancy Carlton, Vice President

Alabama, Florida, Georgia

Southern Division
2 Hanover Square
434 Fayetteville Square Mall, Suite 1650
Raleigh, NC 27601
919-743-5400
Edward L. Owens, Vice President

Kentucky, North Carolina, South Carolina, Tennessee,
Virginia

Western Division
2720 Gateway Oaks Drive, Suite 110
Sacramento, CA 95833
916-924-3232
Michael Clinkenbeard, Vice President

California, Nevada

RECORD BOOK

	12AM	1	2	3	4	5	6	7	8	9	10	11	12PM	1	2	3	4	5	6	7	8	9	10	11
Blood Sugar																								
Meal Bolus																								
High BG Bolus																								
Carbohydrates																								
Fat																								
Urine Ketones																								
Exercise																								
Set Change																								
Basal Rate																								

Comments:

Index

About the American Diabetes Association

The American Diabetes Association is the nation's leading voluntary health organization supporting diabetes research, information, and advocacy. Its mission is to prevent and cure diabetes and to improve the lives of all people affected by diabetes. The American Diabetes Association is the leading publisher of comprehensive diabetes information. Its huge library of practical and authoritative books for people with diabetes covers every aspect of self-care—cooking and nutrition, fitness, weight control, medications, complications, emotional issues, and general self-care.

To order American Diabetes Association books: Call 1-800-232-6733. http://store.diabetes.org [Note: there is no need to use **www** when typing this particular Web address]

To join the American Diabetes Association: Call 1-800-806-7801. www.diabetes.org/membership

For more information about diabetes or ADA programs and services: Call 1-800-342-2383. E-mail: Customerservice@diabetes.org www.diabetes.org

To locate an ADA/NCQA Recognized Provider of quality diabetes care in your area: www.ncqa.org/dprp/

To find an ADA Recognized Education Program in your area: Call 1-888-232-0822. www.diabetes.org/recognition/education.asp

To join the fight to increase funding for diabetes research, end discrimination, and improve insurance coverage: Call 1-800-342-2383. www.diabetes.org/advocacy

To find out how you can get involved with the programs in your community: Call 1-800-342-2383. See below for program Web addresses.

- *American Diabetes Month:* Educational activities aimed at those diagnosed with diabetes—month of November. www.diabetes.org/ADM
- *American Diabetes Alert:* Annual public awareness campaign to find the undiagnosed—held the fourth Tuesday in March. www.diabetes.org/alert
- *The Diabetes Assistance & Resources Program (DAR):* diabetes awareness program targeted to the Latino community. www.diabetes.org/DAR
- *African American Program:* diabetes awareness program targeted to the African American community. www.diabetes.org/africanamerican
- *Awakening the Spirit: Pathways to Diabetes Prevention & Control:* diabetes awareness program targeted to the Native American community. www.diabetes.org/awakening

To find out about an important research project regarding type 2 diabetes: www.diabetes.org/ada/research.asp

To obtain information on making a planned gift or charitable bequest: Call 1-888-700-7029. www.diabetes.org/ada/plan.asp

To make a donation or memorial contribution: Call 1-800-342-2383. www.diabetes.org/ada/cont.asp